The Voice in Ec

The Voice in Education

Vocal Health and Effective Communication

STEPHANIE MARTIN
and
LYN DARNLEY

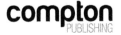

This edition first published 2019 © 2019 by Compton Publishing Ltd.

Registered office: Compton Publishing Ltd, 30 St. Giles',
                                      Oxford, OX1 3LE, UK
Registered company number: 07831037

Editorial offices: 35 East Street, Braunton, EX33 2EA, UK
                                      Web: www.comptonpublishing.co.uk

ISBN 978-1-909082-04-57-1

A catalogue record for this book is available from the British Library.

Cover design: David Siddall, http://www.davidsiddall.com

Set in Adobe Caslon Pro/Myriad Pro 10pt by Stuart Brown

1   2018

Table of Contents

Acknowledgements

The Voice in Education draws not only on the authors' knowledge and practical experience of education but also the generous input from a number of people. The authors would like to thank all those who over the years have offered them guidance and support and to record specific thanks to those within the teaching profession who continue to fulfil such an important role for current and future generations.

In particular, the authors would like to thank Ayesha Ahmed, Jill Boyles, Lindsay Brown, Brian Darnley, Rob Day, Phyliddia Furse, Glenda Goddard-Gill, Lesley Hendy, Janet Hislop, Mary Johnson, Myra Lockhart, Glyn MacDonald, Noel McPherson, Peter Martin, Neil Mercer, Shelley Sawers, Bridget Shield, Heather Steed, Jonathan Stocker, Steve Tasker, Jenn Ward, Hannah Wright, and The British Voice Association.

Preface

This book is intended principally for occupational and professional voice users; individuals, particularly teachers, lecturers, facilitators, and trainers who use their voice for the purposes of education to groups, both large and small, both indoors and outdoors, in a variety of different settings; some of which have little amplification and are vocally very challenging.

Given the changing face of initial teacher training (ITT), prospective teachers and lecturers will come to their role with a variety of previous life experience and pedagogic skills. The aim of this book is to offer information and practical work that allows occupational voice users a mix of easily assimilated theory and practice and strategies for dealing with vocal issues. It is also important to recognise, build, and underpin the transferable skills of those using this book.

The text adopts an integrated approach and offers detailed information on the subject of occupational voice and the vocal demands of the voice user, but also provides detailed information on the physiology of voice and voice care. Practical advice on aspects of clarity of delivery, communication skills, pedagogic skills, and classroom strategies, supported by exercises for developing the above, are provided. In addition, aspects such as the changing teaching environment, acoustic influences on the voice, illness, stress, and anxiety, the ageing voice are explored. Specific qualitative changes such as resonance, as well as range and projection of the voice are included, as are anecdotal personal experiences and challenges from those working in the field. The nature of the work is such that fundamental information is reinforced from a different perspective in a number of chapters.

While not intending to replace professional one-to-one guidance, it is hoped that the book will offer readers strategies, solutions, and tried and tested practical exercises that will enhance their current skills and provide a framework to keep them in good voice throughout their professional careers. The book also includes a number of class-based practical exercises and suggestions for voice, language and communication work with learners and students from age five to 18. These exercises focus on ideas designed to promote spoken English from simple language games to presentation skills and debating. Containing a number of 'at-a-glance' checklists throughout the text and a content section at the end of each chapter, it is hoped that readers will find it an easily accessible resource.

Note on terms used:

'Educators', 'teachers', 'lecturers', and 'trainers' are used interchangeably in the text.

'Learners' is used to denote children from 5 to 15 and 'students' refers to the 16+ age group.

British English pronunciation is used, although it is acknowledged that pronunciation may differ in other accents.

Introduction

What happens when individuals can no longer effectively, inspire, educate, encourage, explore, exchange ideas or concepts, or entertain through the medium of voice?

It is these individuals who have contributed over the past three decades to our joint research and practice. The common foundation of which is an intimate understanding of the anatomy and physiology of the vocal apparatus. Our aim in this book is to carefully consider emotional, physical, ergonomic, environmental, and psychosocial factors and their effect on the voice. Thus we hope to accompany the individual along a journey to rediscover and re-claim the voice they have lost through circumstance, illness, trauma, or misuse, so that they can express themselves with passion and vocal authenticity, maintaining and improving their skills. Additionally, newly qualified teachers, those in training and other occupational voice users can enter, re-enter, and continue in the educational arena with confidence.

The 'Art' of Voice as we see it, relies on a combination of science and art, strongly harnessed by practical work, which allows us to scaffold our approach, using the building bricks of knowledge, recognition, safety, and eclecticism.

This first chapter offers both a framework in which to understand the vulnerability of educators to vocal issues and the socio-political environment within which they function. Exercises in isolation and without context fail, in our opinion, to appropriately address the effect of the constellation of issues faced by educators.

An efficient and effective voice is an essential requirement for teachers, lecturers, and trainers. Teaching, as Lemov (2016) suggests, is a performance profession so it would be difficult to imagine working proficiently in such a profession without this most important working tool.

Teachers, lecturers, trainers, and facilitators (referred to collectively as educators) are known as professional and occupational voice users. This generic term also applies to actors, politicians, radio announcers, barristers, the clergy, telesales workers, singers, and facilitators. Voice is a critical factor of all these professional roles and continued employment is therefore dependent on maintaining vocal effectiveness through diligent vocal care and conservation.

The last thirty years have seen an increase in the attention paid to both the prevention and management of voice disorders in the workplace and the effective delivery of information, but despite the number of individuals whose living is dependent on training and maintenance of the voice, this critical 'working tool', still remains under-resourced. While the focus of this book lies with the vocal care, maintenance, and performance needs of teachers, lecturers, and trainers, the information it provides applies equally to *all* professional voice users.

As with other 'on the job' training, a reasonable expectation would be that as voice use is a critical component of the professional/educational role, training would be available to bring vocal skills up to a 'professional' level, but regrettably this is not the case. 'Professional' suggests a level of vocal expertise, ability, and training that allows individuals to use their voice effectively in a variety of settings and to different groups and numbers of people. In the case of 'professional' or 'occupational' voice users, however, the term is more often used to denote the amount of time during their working day that they spend talking, in other words the 'vocal loading' they experience, rather than any voice training that has been offered or undertaken.

Despite the availability of electronic teaching aids and devices, 'vocal loading', remains of considerable concern for teachers, lecturers, and trainers. Some years ago Martin (2003), reported that newly qualified teachers and lecturers in their first year in post were talking for over 60 per cent of each teaching session, representing very high vocal demand and subsequently high vocal loading. In the case of those working within primary education this was consistently at high volume, whereas for those within further or higher education a more balanced use of high and medium volume was reported.

Levels of vocal usage and loading

Little has changed over the past decades. Koufman first identified levels of vocal usage in 1998, showing a link between professional demands and vocal load, and her categorization below remains cogent and current today.

- The Elite Vocal Performer, Level I, is a person for who even a slight aberration of voice may have dire consequences. Most singers and actors would fall into this group, with the opera singer representing the quintessential Level I performer.
- *The Professional Voice User, Level II*, is a person for whom a moderate vocal problem might prevent adequate job performance. Here, Koufman would include teachers, lecturers, politicians, and the clergy. (Italics are the authors').
- The Non-Vocal Professional, Level III, is categorized as a person for whom a severe vocal problem would prevent adequate job performance. This group includes lawyers, physicians, and businessmen and women.
- The Non-Vocal Professional, Level IV, is a person for whom vocal quality is not a prerequisite for adequate job performance. In this group would be found, for example, labourers and office staff.

Studies in the National Centre for Voice and Speech (NCVS), at the University of Utah, (Hunter and Titze, 2010) compared the vocal demands placed on teachers through the comparison of their occupational voice use with their non-occupational voice use. In Hunter and Titze's study occupational voice use was designated as from 9 AM–3 PM and non-occupational voice use as from 4 PM–10 PM, plus weekends. Fifty-seven were in the study and key factors emerged to show that:

- Previous findings of occupational (~30%) and non-occupational voicing (14%) were substantiated.
- Teachers experienced a wide range of occupational voicing percentages (33%, SD ±11%).

- Occupational voice use was on average only about 1 decibel (dB) louder than non-occupational voice and remained constant through-out the day.
- Occupational voice exhibited a higher pitch, increasing upwards throughout the day.

Vulnerability of educators to voice problems

Studies over the past thirty years confirm a consistently high worldwide inci-dence of voice problems within the teaching population in comparison to other occupations.

- Occupational or professional voice users form a disproportionately large number of patients attending for voice therapy. Twenty years ago, Morton and Watson (1998) reported that in Northern Ireland, teachers made up 15% of the patient case load, yet only 2% of the total workforce. Over a decade ago in the United States, studies reported a figure of 20% of the patient caseload (Roy *et al.* 2004).
- Teachers are reported as absent from work due to voice problems twice as often as others in vocally demanding professions (De Jong *et al.*, 2006).
- In Spain, Preciado-Lopez *et al.* (2008) reported 3.87 new cases per year per one thousand teachers.
- Lockhart's unpublished 2008 audit showed that 20% of the voice case load in Lanarkshire, Scotland were teachers.

A longitudinal study in the United Kingdom, (Martin, 2003), showed that, in a sample of 50 prospective teachers:

- Only 54% presented with a vocal quality which, on perceptual voice quality rating, was considered to 'be within normal limits'.
- 30% presented with a vocal quality that was considered to be of slight concern.
- 16% presented with a vocal quality that was of definite concern.

- 77% of the student teacher cohort, who were about to begin a six
  week initial teaching placement and whose vocal quality was considered 'vulnerable', experienced changes in voice quality after completing the placement.

A much larger study conducted in Sweden by Ohlsson *et al.* (2012) on
1250 prospective teacher students reported that 17% of the students had voice
problems defined as at least two symptoms weekly.

A significant feature of both these studies is that, as the students were at
the beginning of their studies and had not yet been exposed to teaching practice, risk factors were individual rather than being affected by their working
environment. It is recognized that both genetic and environmental factors
may cause voice disorders, so given the large percentage of students already
demonstrating voice problems in the studies above (Martin, 2003; Ohlsson
et al., 2012), the heavy vocal demands of the teaching role, cannot have failed
to add to the potential for further vocal risk to those students.

This vocal risk was confirmed by the number of those in Martin's study
(2003) who experienced vocal change during the first term of teaching and
the fact that all within the sample reported that they had experienced vocal
change at some point. In the same study, the voice quality of the same cohort
of teachers was compared and contrasted at a later stage in their careers when
it was found that 79% of voices were considered to have some degree of alteration after two years of teaching.

While it would not be deemed appropriate to select prospective teacher
students on the basis of the health of their vocal folds, given the implications of the studies above it would seem that more attention to a pre-training
assessment of prospective teachers' vocal robustness might be advisable.

Occupational health issues

Studies consistently demonstrate the negative effect on the voice of prolonged
speaking without proper training and the subsequent adverse impact on professional careers and employers due to days lost. Almost a quarter of a cen-

tury has passed since litigation was taken in the UK by Clowry (1992), and Oldfield (1994) and in the past decade by Walters, (Hazards, 2010), which highlight the vocal problems experienced by those in the teaching profession. The courts found in favour of the teachers, whose voice loss, which effectively forced them into early retirement, was agreed to be due to the demands of their teaching roles. It is to be regretted that given the occupational health directives below, the evidence from these cases still do not appear to have led to a review of the way in which voice care and training is delivered as part of a national drive to prevent vocal attrition among teachers.

- As long ago as 1974 in the United Kingdom the Health and Safety at Work Act required employers to do 'all that is reasonably practical to safeguard the health, safety, and welfare of their employees at work'.

- A Europe-wide survey on Occupational Safety and Health (OS&H) *Arrangements for Voice and Speech Professionals* (Vilkman, 2000; 2004) recorded responses from 15 countries. Vilkman noted that, using OS&H legislation as a background for the professional voice user, there is a poor level of application of the 1989 Council Directive entitled 'On the introduction of measures to encourage improvements in the safety and health of workers at work'.[1] This directive deals, among others, with such issues as the prevention of occupational risks and the protection of safety and health.

- It took until 2005 in the United Kingdom for teaching unions to warn education employers to change archaic working conditions that were causing voice loss and other health problems.

- In 2006, the United Kingdom Industrial Injuries Advisory Council (IIAC, 2006) carried out a review of the literature on occupational voice loss, but the Council found it was not possible to identify a condition with unique clinical features specifically associated with prolonged heavy vocal use stating, there was a 'lack of good qual-

---

1   Directive 89/391/EEC – OSH "Framework Directive" of 12 June 1989, European Agency for Safety and Health at Work.

ity epidemiological data'. This finding was extremely discouraging considering the number of studies, linking teaching demands and voice problems.

- More encouraging, however, is the redefinition in the United Kingdom of the terms of the Disability Discrimination Act in 2010. This means that people with medical conditions which are controlled but could still recur, such as a voice disorder, are now covered by the act.

In the United States, The Gallup-Healthways Well-Being Index (Forbes, 2013) surveyed 94,000 workers across 14 major occupations in the U.S. Of the 77% of workers who fit the survey's definition of having a chronic health condition (asthma, cancer, depression, diabetes, heart attack, high blood pressure, high cholesterol, or obesity), to which, although not stated, could be added voice loss, the total annual costs relating to lost productivity totalled $84 billion. According to the survey, the annual costs associated with absenteeism in the teaching profession amounted to $5.6 billion. As will be explored later in this book, teachers are at risk of absenteeism not only due to voice loss but also for any or all of the reasons below as cited by Forbes:

- Bullying and harassment – employees who are bullied or harassed by co-workers and/or bosses are more likely to call in sick to avoid the situation.
- Burnout, stress, and low morale – heavy workloads, stressful meetings/presentations, and feelings of being unappreciated can cause employees to avoid going into work. Personal stress (outside of work) can lead to absenteeism.
- Depression – according to the National Institute of Mental Health, the leading cause of absenteeism in the United States is depression. Depression can also lead to substance abuse if people turn to drugs or alcohol to self-medicate their pain or anxiety.
- Disengagement – employees who are not committed to their jobs, co-workers, and/or the company or institution are more likely to miss work simply because they have no motivation to attend

- Illness – injuries, illness, and medical appointments are the most commonly reported reasons for missing work (though not always the actual reason).
- Injuries – accidents can occur on the job or outside of work, resulting in absences. In addition to acute injuries, chronic injuries such as back and neck problems are a common cause of absenteeism.

In the United States, information from the University of Iowa (2017) stated that working on the evidence of a study by Dr. Katherine Verdolini and Dr. Lorraine Ramig, the cost of teachers' voice problems on an annual basis was $2.5 billion. This figure included medical costs, pharmacy, and insurance expenses plus substitute teacher costs.

Teachers are about 4% of the U.S. workforce, yet are almost 20% of the patient load in voice clinics. Given that at the time there were 5,168,000 U.S. teachers, of which approximately 40% experience voice problems, that would seem to indicate that 2,067,200 teachers have hoarseness, fatigue, or other voice difficulties. Of that group, only 15% actually sought treatment. Similarly, in the United Kingdom, many fewer teachers who experience voice loss, report a problem or seek treatment.

References

Clowry P. 1996. *The Times* Letters, 30 December 1996.

De Jong FICRS, Kooijman PGC, Thomas G, Huinck, *et al*. 2006. Epidemiology of voice problems in Dutch Teachers. *Folia Phoniatrica et Logopaedica* **58**: 186–98.

Hazards. 2010. Available at: <www.hazards.org/voiceloss/voicelessons.htm> [Accessed August 2017].

Health and Safety at Work Act 1974. Available at: <http://www.hse.gov.uk/legislation/hswa.htm> [Accessed August 2017].

Hunter EJ, Titze IR. 2010. Variations in intensity, fundamental frequency and voicing for teachers in occupational versus non occupational settings. *Journal of Speech, Language, Hearing Research* **53**: 862–75.

Industrial Injuries Advisory Council. 2006. Available at: <www.iiac.org.uk> [Accessed August 2017].

Koufman JA. 1998. Available at: <http://www.speechpathology.com/articles/what-voice-disorders-and-who-1508-1508> [Accessed August 2017].

Lemov D. 2010. *Teach like a Champion*. San Francisco, CA: Jossey-Bass.

Lockhart M. 2008. *The Breathing and Voice Workout*. Unpublished exercise programme.

Martin S. 2003. An exploration of factors which have an impact on the vocal performance and vocal effectiveness of newly qualified teachers/lecturers. PhD thesis, University of Greenwich.

Morton V and Watson DR. 1998. The teaching voice: problems and perceptions. *Logopedics Phoniatrics Vocology* 23: 133–9.

Morton V and Watson DR. 2001. The impact of impaired vocal quality on children's ability to process spoken language. *Logopedics Phoniatrics Vocology* 26(1): 17–25.

Ohlsson AC, Andersson EM, Sodersten M, *et al.* 2012. Prevalence of voice symptoms and risk factor in teacher students. *Journal of Voice* 26(5): 629–34.

Oldfield P. 1995. *PAT Fact Sheet* (Professional Association of Teachers).

Preciado-Lopez J, Perez-Fernandez C, Calzada-Uriondo M, and Preciado-Ruiz P. 2008. Epidemiological study of voice disorders among teaching professionals of La Rioja, Spain. *Journal of Voice* 22(4) : 489–508.

Roy N, Merrill RM, Thibeault S, and Smith EM. 2004. Voice disorders in teachers and the general population: effects on work performance, attendance and future career choices. *Journal of Speech, Language and Hearing Research* 47: 542–51.

Roy N, Merill RM, Thibeault S, *et al.* 2004 Prevalence of voice disorders in teachers and general population. *Journal of Voice* 47: 281–93.

University of Iowa. 2017. Available at: <https://uiowa.edu/voice-academy/numbers-dont-lie> [Accessed August 2017].

Vilkman, E. 2000. Voice problems at work: A challenge for occupational safety and health arrangement. *Folia Phoniatrica et Logopaedica* 52: 120–5.

Vilkman, E. 2004. Occupational safety and health aspects of voice and speech professions. *Folia Phoniatrica et Logopaedica* 56: 220–53.

1

The teacher, lecturer, and trainer as a professional voice user

The role of voice in the communication process

Vocal quality is accepted as an essential parameter of the communication process and a voice disorder compromises the effectiveness of the message. The communication process is, by its very nature, a transactional process. What takes place when two or more people interact is underpinned by a constellation of perceptual, cognitive, affective, and performative factors (Hargie, 2006).

Models of communication have existed for many years, both earlier and later than that of Shannon and Weaver's (1949) communication model of almost seven decades ago in which they examined the communication process between two individuals. They proposed that one individual was designated as the Source, the other as the Receiver. Their thinking at that time was that the Source transmitted a message to the Receiver. Communication models now suggest that communicators are at one and the same time both senders and receivers of messages. The Source, while monitoring the effects of his/her utterance, is at the same time a Receiver, as he/she acquires feedback from the Receiver. Likewise the Receiver, in listening to the Source, is also reacting to the Source's contribution even if only to ignore it. Each individual in the communication process is in fact a 'source-receiver'.

Communication is ubiquitous; it appears to be everywhere and ever present (Dickson *et al.*, 1989). The exponential increase in digital communication during the past three decades confirms this statement, but Dickson *et al.* could not have predicted that this increase has, in effect, altered the balance between verbal and non-verbal communication (reducing the verbal and increasing the written element of communication). Voice is one component of interpersonal communication and is of considerable importance to professional voice users, as voice contributes to the effectiveness of the process by which information, meaning, and feelings are shared through the exchange of verbal messages. The increased and increasing use of digital communication has, in truth, the potential to reduce the skill set of those for whom voice is a major signifier of performative factors in communication, underlining the importance of additional training for those professional voice users who have less than robust vocal technique.

In its simplest form the communication process has been identified as including:

- The communicators (which have been discussed above).
- The message – which needs to be made known, encoded, or organized into a physical form capable of being transmitted to others. Decoding is the counterpart of encoding, whereby recipients attach meaning to what they have just experienced.
- The medium – which is the particular way of conveying the message and here, voice is a critical medium with which to convey the message.
- The channel – in verbal exchanges communicators use the vocal-auditory channel which carries speech.
- The noise – in communication terms, noise refers to any interference with the success of the communicative act or distortion of the message, so that the meaning is not understood.

- The feedback – judging the extent of how successfully the message has been received and the impact it has had on the listener is through feedback.
- The context – all communication takes place within a context and the context is crucially important for the success or otherwise of the communication. The time, relationship, and geography of the exchange exerts considerable influence on the success or otherwise of such.

Looking at the role of voice in the communication process (outlined above) it can be seen that a voice disorder would compromise the effectiveness of the message in all categories, namely the message, the medium, the channel, the noise, the feedback, and the context. Three seminal studies (McSporran, 1997; Morton and Watson, 2001; Rogerson and Dodd, 2005) have shown the effect of a teacher's voice disorder on students' learning. McSporran noted that children taught by teachers with voice problems potentially learn less well, while Rogerson and Dodd showed that impaired voice placed additional demands on the listener as more resources are directed to perceptual processing, thus reducing processing capacity for the understanding of information. The importance of verbal and non-verbal communication is explored in further detail in Chapter 7.

Voice care and training provision

For the majority of voice patients, voice therapy is usually successful and treatment options are predicated on evidence-based therapy. Preventative voice care should therefore be successful in mitigating the worst effects of vocal damage. As a consequence of preventative training, teachers, lecturers, and trainers should be better able to monitor and sustain their own voice effectively throughout their working life, leading to a reduction in the number of those experiencing problems.

It is important to stress that it is not the case that teachers, lecturers, and trainers would never experience voice problems if they were to have training.

For a small number of vocally vulnerable individuals voice problems could still occur. It is not possible to disregard the contribution of lifelong speech habits, such as the tendency to speak rapidly, excessively, and/or loudly, to the 'wear and tear' of the vocal mechanism. It is, however, likely that with preventative voice work the risk would be limited and/or diminished.

While accepting those variables, training teachers in voice care can be demonstrated to have a beneficial preventive effect on subsequent vocal damage. Studies such as those of Ohlsson *et al.* (2016) have demonstrated that despite extensive dropout from their randomized control trial, voice education for teacher students has a preventive effect.

Requirements issued to all training institutions in the UK by the Department for Education in 1992 stated that, among other things, all qualified teachers must be able to communicate clearly and effectively through questioning, instructing, explaining, and feedback (DfE, 1992). This continued to be part of the updated Circulars issued by the Department for Education and Skills (DfES). New standards and requirements included in 'Qualifying to Teach' (TTA, 2002), which apply to all trainee teachers and programmes of initial teacher training in England from September 2002, state that those awarded qualified teacher status must demonstrate that they can 'communicate sensitively and effectively with parents and carers' (TPU 0803/02-02).

In March 2016, a Government White Paper was published which stated that teachers in the United Kingdom will have to prove that they can handle naughty children in the classroom before taking up the profession, and the Qualified Teacher Status will be replaced with a more challenging test. Aspriring teachers will only be qualified once they have demonstrated classroom proficiency, including behaviour management. The DfE has recently released four documents for Initial Teacher Training (ITT) which include *Behaviour Management* and *ITT Core Content*. Dr Lesley Hendy, one of the authors of 'Five Main Voices for Effective Teaching' (Hendy and Parke, 2015), presented information about their work to the DfE, but the only mention of voice that appears to have made it into the new documents was in the *Behaviour Management* document, where it received one brief mention under a section called 'Normalizing good behaviour and reducing attention misbehaviour'. This read as follows: Body Language, voice tone, language choice (p. 11).

There was considerable disappointment amongst those working with teachers, lecturers, and trainers that little mention was made of the importance of voice in helping with behaviour management, as well as the essential role voice plays in delivering information. As has been already noted in this chapter, vocal attrition compromises the effectiveness of the message and a teacher's voice problem can affect pupils' education.

A more consistent and targeted approach to voice care in teacher training is still awaited, despite initiatives from General Teaching Councils in Northern Ireland, Scotland, and Wales. The General Teaching Council for Scotland produced a policy document about voice in the teaching profession. The DfES, in their Healthy Schools, Healthy Teachers (2001) website, recommends that teachers and trainee teachers should be referred to specialist help from a speech and language therapist and/or an ear, nose, and throat (ENT) consultant should they experience vocal problems.

Vocal requirements for teaching

If teachers are to teach effectively, the undisputed fact is that they need voices that are able to withstand the demands of prolonged voice use, often at high volume, on a daily basis (Martin, 2003). Research completed between 2000 and 2012 in the United States at The National Centre for Voice and Speech (NCVS) into occupational voice use has quantified damage–risk for teachers, and they have set a 30% damage–risk criterion for the combination of three variables – loudness, duration, and fundamental frequency – paralleling research on damage–risk for hearing loss. These factors are explored in more detail below.

It is possible to use the voice for prolonged periods of time, without tiring, damaging, or abusing it, but for all but the most vocally robust this requires prior training in, for example:

- How to use and care for the voice effectively and efficiently.
- How to manage and monitor the voice in less than ideal conditions.
- How to manage the voice in physically and/or emotionally challenging situations.

Few, if any, teachers work in ideal conditions. Ideal conditions in terms of physical space would be acoustically balanced, warm but not overheated, well-ventilated buildings. Few teachers are able to produce and sustain vocal quality and volume in an easy and relaxed manner with well balanced posture, good control of breath, and minimal mental stress over a long period. Factors that contribute to this less than ideal vocal environment are discussed below.

Physical challenges of the classroom setting

Classroom noise

Noise is a consistent and relatively well recognized vocal health risk factor in teachers' working environments. Noise levels in the classroom place considerable demands on teachers' voices and thereby increase the vocal loading. The Department for Education in England upgraded guidelines for environmental design in schools (The Stationery Office, 1997) but before that date there was no information on acceptable noise levels in school classrooms. Smythe and Bamford's study (1997) looked at speech perception of four primary age hearing-impaired children in mainstream classrooms in the UK, suggesting that there should be up-to-date information on classroom acoustics and hearing ability at all levels. Improving acoustic conditions for hearing-impaired children in mainstream schools benefits the listening conditions for all children and, as a result, has advantages in reduced stress and vocal effort for teachers.

Current thinking in education is to encourage children to verbalize ideas and explore language so that they can use speech to explore their world and develop their social and personal skills. This is particularly important given the recent information emerging from a 'State of Education' (2016) report by The Key regarding the level of language skills with which small children enter school. Almost a third of four-year-olds (at least 194,000 children) were not considered to be ready for the classroom as they were said to lack the speech, language, and communication skills needed to cope when they start school.

'School leaders are already struggling to retain staff and manage their teachers' workload, so add thousands more pupils arriving ill-prepared to the equation and the burden placed on our schools will be huge' said Fergal Roche, CEO of The Key.

These findings should be seen in relation to the burden it places on the teacher's voice, as the teacher's desire is to make sure that children with limited language experience can not only understand but also clearly hear his/her voice in order to learn. In an effort to ensure that children can hear their teachers' voices well over background noise, teachers tend to raise their vocal volume, perhaps more than necessary or in a compensatory way. Many teachers' voices just cannot sustain that high daily vocal burden.

While many children are more skilled at swiping a tablet than communicating vocally, young children are not, for the most part, programmed to sustain long periods without talking and indeed, anecdotal reports suggest that a similar situation exists in secondary, further, and higher education. At all levels within education, group assignments and presentations are increasingly used to examine academic performance. In September 2015 students in the UK began studying a new General Certificate of Secondary Education (GCSE) in English Language (graded 9 to 1) for the first award in 2017. The GCSE exams (formerly known as O-levels) were introduced in 1988 and are single-subject exams taken upon completion of two years of study at the age of 16 (age at US 10th grade). Students take anywhere between five and 10 subjects which, if passed, are generally considered equivalent to a US high school diploma. This new English Language GCSE is based on new subject content, including the requirement that students are assessed on their ability to demonstrate their spoken language skills. This additional assessment is to be welcomed in terms of increased oracy skills in pupils, but in terms of voice conservation, it may be less welcome to the teacher, as there are few periods in the day when vocalization without competing background noise occurs.

'Training' and reviewing student practice for this additional assessment will patently increase the teacher's vocal loading. It is therefore most important that the teacher develops pedagogical strategies to maximize opportunities for easy voicing.

Educators, particularly the newly qualified, may find it difficult to assess the degree of vocal effort needed to be heard over a particular level of background noise, often reporting that their voice was unequal to the task. This increased effort can lead to early episodes of vocal strain. An unfortunate consequence of vocal strain early in one's professional life is that although periods of vocal rest away from school will help to ease the problem (which is why teachers often report that holiday periods help to alleviate the symptoms), once a pattern has been established it is difficult for the teacher to alter voice use without help. The teacher, lecturer, or trainer returns to work and the voice problem returns. Finding help from an outside agency once voice problems are present may be difficult to access or arrange, which is why training before the educator goes into the teaching environment is so essential.

Classroom design

Even when background noise is not a problem, classroom design is often ill thought out in terms of the demands that it places on the teacher's voice and with the safe use of teachers' voices in mind. New schools are built to encourage openness, which is invaluable in terms of the school functioning as a community, but using the voice effectively without training in large open spaces is not always easy. In their 2015 study, Durup *et al.* reported:

> The requirement for appropriately low noise levels and suitable intelligibility in teaching rooms in now widely acknowledged as being essential for effective pupil learning. However, to date less attention has been given to the needs of teachers and the impact of poor acoustic design on the teacher's voice.

The structure of buildings and the materials used inside them determine their ultimate acoustic quality:

- In general, low ceilings, carpeted floors, covered walls, and soft furnishings tend to 'dampen and deaden' sound and consequently absorb the voice. This dampening and deadening of sound is generally true of most primary and elementary schools, where there are numerous artifacts on the walls and ceilings which have been fashioned by the children.
- Hard surfaces, such as varnished timber or wooden tiles, steel-framed windows and doors, large expanses of glass, and bare walls, tend to produce a bright, sharp, and occasionally echoing sound.

A good acoustic environment provides conditions in which noise is suppressed and speech is clear and words are easily distinguishable.

Working in new, purpose-built, high-tech schools with lots of glass, exposed brickwork, and open spaces is often just as demanding vocally as working in older schools. Older schools, which range from those housed in their original nineteenth century buildings with cathedral roofs to the glass and concrete structures of the 1960s, all have their own problems acoustically and environmentally, and these should not be overlooked. The effect on the voice of the acoustic space is very important to the teacher. Primary school teachers often spend their whole day teaching in one space; teachers and lecturers in the secondary and tertiary sectors find that they have to work in a variety of spaces.

World Health Organization (WHO) guidelines (2001) recommend a noise level of 35 dB(A) for school classrooms during lessons to avoid disturbance of communication. Actually, noise levels in schools frequently exceed these limits and can reach as much as 60–80 dB(A) in normal classes; they can even go beyond limit values for workplaces in school workshops and sports areas. Studies from the European Agency for Safety and Health at Work, looking at noise in education, reported on measurements in several classrooms in everyday use which revealed acoustical conditions that permit less than half of the speech to be understood. Generally, the problems were caused by improper wall, ceiling, and floor finishes, and by noisy ventilation equipment.

The effect of trying to compete with an acoustically difficult environment creates a problem of severe vocal strain for many teachers.

It is encouraging, however, to note an increasing awareness within education of the importance of the teaching environment. While there have been building design guidance documents on school acoustics for many decades (Shield, 2011), new school buildings in England and Wales became subject to building regulations for the first time in 2003. A new edition, The Building Regulations &c. (Amendment) Regulations 2015, contains updated requirements for acoustics in educational spaces.

Shield *et al.* (2015) made an extensive survey of acoustic conditions in secondary schools which highlighted the importance of good acoustic design to achieve good speaking and learning conditions in classrooms. In particular, relationships between lesson noise levels and unoccupied acoustic conditions emphasize the necessity of considering the acoustic conditions in all teaching spaces in a school at the design stage of a building or its refurbishment. The acoustic design should aim to reduce the unoccupied noise levels and reverberation times to minimize noise levels during lessons and to optimize acoustic conditions for teaching and learning.

Similarly, classrooms are principally arranged to accommodate the needs of the learners and students, rather than providing for the vocal and ergonomic needs of the teacher. A combination of hard and soft surfaces designed to suit the space can help greatly, while acoustic professionals can be brought in to help alleviate some of the acoustic difficulties.

Educators working in large spaces, such as lecture rooms and large classrooms, encounter problems related to the natural loss of sound over distance:

- At a distance of 6 m, sounds are only a quarter as strong as they were at a distance of 3 m.
- At 12 m they are only a little over a twentieth as strong as they were at 3 m.

For many teachers and lecturers, the problems of teaching a class in a large space is one of attempting to 'reach' those at the back without too much vocal effort. If educators are unable to modify their 'teaching' voice to accommodate the variable acoustics, given noise variances etc. of the space, then they will, for the most part, attempt to counteract the effect by potentially vocally abusive behaviours such as pushing or straining the voice or increasing the volume. Durup *et al.* (2015) shows a positive correlation between internal ambient noise levels in classrooms and the speech levels of teachers working in those rooms. The study noted that the higher the internal ambient level, the higher the teacher's speech level, thus highlighting the potential for a greater risk of voice problems for teachers working in those classrooms or lecture halls.

For those who find themselves working in such an environment, it is helpful to 'choreograph' the space, so that they can determine how to move within it, using Lemov's acronym SCAT (Specific, Concrete, Actionable, Techniques) to think of ways to circumvent the acoustic challenges of the classroom.

Lemov (2010) talks of techniques which he cumulatively calls Strong Voice (although his taxonomy of voice is different to that used in this publication), and in acoustically challenging situations they offer a way of reducing vocal output and effort while maintaining control.

His five principles, while designed to be used in interactions with learners and students to 'command' authority, also allow for a reduction in vocal output and effort. They are as follows:

- **Economy of language.** Lemov advocates demonstrating economy of language through the use of fewer words, using words that best focus on what is important, avoid initiating distractions and excess words in the classroom.
- **Do not talk over.** Lemov advocates waiting until there is no other talking or rustling, ensuring that your voice never competes for attention. Controlling the floor is a mark of authority.
- **Do not engage.** Once the topic of conversation is set, avoid engaging in other topics of conversation, refuse to engage with students who want to hijack the class's attention.
- **Square up/stand still.** Non-verbal communication is as important

as verbal so Lemov recommends positioning (both shoulders and feet) directly opposite the learner or student to whom you are speaking, stop and don't engage in other tasks at the same time as giving directions.

- **Quiet power.** Get slower and quieter when you want control, lower your voice and students will strain to listen. Do not get louder or faster.

Chapters 6, 7, and 9 explore strategies for educators that are effective in limiting vocal strain within their working environment, offering suggestions for working with, rather than against, the demands of their environment, and suggestions for mitigating the effects of stress and anxiety on the voice. In Chapters 10, 11, and 12, readers will find exercises for volume, pitch, clarity, projection, relaxation, and posture.

Classroom ergonomics

In early years classes children sit on small chairs around small tables - a seating plan that is designed to encourage conversation and to give the small child security and a feeling of being at home in a friendly environment. This is obviously important in terms of creating a positive learning environment, but it offers unlimited opportunities for the children to talk among themselves, thus increasing the level of background noise over which the teacher has to speak. It also places increased strain on the vocal mechanism because the height of the tables means that the teacher, in order to make eye contact when talking to the learners, has either to crouch by the side of the table or to bend over.

The following chapter gives information on the anatomy and structure of the larynx and how the voice is affected both directly and indirectly by postural changes, but it is important to stress, at this point, that bending awkwardly and vocalizing at the same time is not conducive to easy voicing (see Figure 1.1). Crouching, although possibly less dignified, is more vocally desirable because it maintains the important head/neck alignment and therefore prevents strain on the external and internal musculature of the larynx (see Figure 1.2). Crouching or bending at the knee requires much more conscious effort than a spontaneous and instinctive bend in response to a small

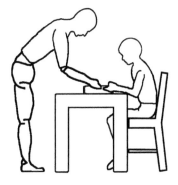 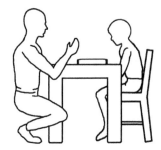

Figure 1.1: Incorrect position.   **Figure 1.2:** Correct position.

learner. That action, however, brings with it concomitant strain on the back, neck, and ultimately the voice.

Actors who are required to perform in physically limiting positions would generally insist on being taught the necessary physical and vocal techniques in order to prevent vocal strain. If necessary, they might involve the support of their union. The same recourse to official support and guidance does not, however, appear to apply to the teaching profession.

Vocal awareness

Commerce, industry, and politics acknowledge the benefit of training in voice and communication skills, yet there do not appear to be the same drivers in education. One reason may be that within the population at large, incidents of voice loss or vocal misuse remain a low priority on the scale of significant illness. This may be due to a lack of awareness or, where there is awareness, what might be described as a rather *laissez-faire* attitude to voice problems.

This attitude appears to have filtered down to education, where there appears to be limited recognition of the vocal demands of teaching and a long term lack of awareness and recognition of the importance and need to train the 'teaching voice'. In addition there seems to be a tacit acceptance that voice problems 'come with the territory' – if you teach you expect to have voice problems. The received wisdom seems to be that these will occur with more or less frequency and be of greater or lesser severity according to 'luck'. You are lucky if you get through a term without a problem. Many teachers do effect temporary improvement through voice rest, although a significant number of teachers experiencing vocal change simply 'put up with it'.

Regrettably, this attitude can lead to a spiral of periodic voice loss, followed by periods of remission as a result of vocal rest, through to a gradual acceptance that perhaps the voice is not as good as it was but it will probably never be any better. Slowly, there is a loss of ability to appraise the voice critically and to notice changes. If proper voice training were given as part of teacher training most teachers would be given the skills to monitor and sustain their own voice effectively throughout their working life. It would also provide a cost-effective solution to a problem which currently costs education authorities considerable sums in lost time and staff replacements.

Vocal dysfunction should not be seen as something to treat as an occasional 'hazard'. Rather, it should be appropriately attributed to the effects of vocal misuse.

Additional vocal challenges

In assessing the vocal demands of the teaching role the extra, vocally-demanding duties that teachers undertake are often forgotten. Responsibilities such as playground duty mean that many teachers end up shouting to gain attention out-of-doors in all weather. Similarly with sports activities, where children are generally noisy and very excited, teachers often have no other recourse than to shout when trying to gain their attention. Shouting under stress, unless done properly through a learned technique, is potentially very vocally abusive. Chapter 10 considers extreme volume in detail.

Sports classes held inside in a gym with little ventilation are also full of vocal 'minefields', but possibly the most difficult situation of all is where a teacher has to supervise learners and students in echoing swimming pools. One teacher remarked that her voice had never been the same since she started to coach swimming at a municipal baths. She simply tried to shout louder to make herself heard and ended up experiencing quite severe vocal strain.

Although there is an acceptance that certain extracurricular activities do require special skills and allowances are given, there are very few occasions on which recommendations are made regarding the vocal skills required. Drama classes, music and singing classes form part of the primary teacher's role; indeed music is an essential component of teaching within the primary school. For many teachers, these vocally-demanding activities prove to be too much and their voices 'break down', sometimes resulting in the need to change profession. Anecdotal comments from teachers report, for example, that they used to be able to sing but now cannot do more than guide and monitor their students – their vocal range has dramatically diminished. Many teachers who have acquired skills in an *ad hoc* manner, as a result of their teaching experience, need additional training to cope with such intense vocal demands.

After school clubs, activities and sporting fixtures place further demands on vocally vulnerable teachers. Not to be seen to play a full and active part in the school by 'volunteering' for these extracurricular activities may be perceived as tantamount to signaling an unwillingness to give full support to the school, or that their interest in promotion or advancement within the profession is limited. **Chapter 9** looks beyond the teaching role and explores some of the additional duties that teachers and lecturers may have to take on as part of their professional role.

Demographic changes in the UK have shown an increase in the school age population over successive years, but a reduction in teacher training entry numbers and teachers leaving the profession as a result of stress and anxiety create severe shortages in teacher:pupil ratios. A survey of 4,500 teachers, carried out by *The Guardian* newspaper (2016), found many teachers across England were at crisis point: 98% said they were under increasing pressure and 82% described their workload as 'unmanageable'. More than three-quarters were working between 49 and 65 hours a week: nearly three-quarters (73%) said their workload was having a serious impact on their physical health, and 75% on their mental health. Only 12% said they have good work–life balance and only a third felt that their employers considered their wellbeing (Lightfoot, 2016).

In the same survey, 79% of schools said they were struggling to recruit or retain teachers, and 88% predicted that things would get worse and that it would severely affect students. Mary Bousted, then General Secretary of the trades union The Association of Teachers and Lecturers (ATL), said their internal records confirm *The Guardian*'s findings: "This is the worst time for teacher recruitment since 2003 when I took up this post" she said. "We know 50,000 teachers left last year, that's 11% of the workforce, and we will have 300,000 more pupils in our schools by 2020. It's largely due to the toxic mix of accountability pressures, curriculum and qualification reform, compounded by mixed messages from the Government" (Lightfoot, 2016).

As has been noted, with fewer teachers in post having to teach increased numbers of pupils, greater pressure is placed on those in work. In this climate, teachers who are vocally vulnerable experience even more pressure at work, adding to their level of stress and anxiety and ultimately their inability to continue in the profession. Teacher recruitment and retention is becoming a growing problem in the teaching profession. The State of Education survey report of 2016 reported that about six in 10 (62%) school leaders found it challenging to recruit and retain teachers. It was a particular challenge for secondary school leaders, with about three-quarters (76%) saying that they found it difficult to manage in their schools compared with just under six in 10 leaders in primary settings (59%).

Dr Lesley Hendy, in a letter to the DfE (2016), part of which is reproduced here with permission from the author, said in relation to the importance of the human voice in teaching and behaviour management: "The country needs qualified, effective teachers who can control a class to provide the maximum opportunity for pupils to learn. Classroom disruption costs the country both in economic and societal terms".

For many years, Dr Lesley Hendy and her colleague Suzanne Parke have been providing voice training for trainee teachers in different parts of the United Kingdom, completing the majority of their work in the county of Essex, with two School-Centred Initial Teacher Training programmes (SCITTs) in particular, those of Thames Primary Consortium and The Essex SCITT.

Both these SCITTs have recorded that the five-year survey of retention rate shows that Thames Primary Consortium has achieved 96% and The Essex SCITT, over 90%. As they note: 'With the national retention rate at 60%, the training we are giving is surely worth researching'. They go on to comment on the cost to education and health of remedial vocal therapy for teachers who have vocal problems, as well as the loss to the profession.

Repetitive strain injury (RSI) has enjoyed considerable attention world-wide and, indeed, has been proved to be a painful and distressing side effect for many workers. Substantial damages have been awarded to those who had suffered RSI and could prove that this had occurred as a function of their working life. Increased attention has now been focused on what could be described as 'RSI of the vocal folds' in terms of occupational voice disorders. What researchers are investigating is the link between the strain imposed on the vocal folds through sustained voicing over long periods and the amount of recovery time that is available to the individual (Titze, 2012). Emerging evidence from call centre personnel shows that many are experiencing significant vocal problems as a result of unremitting vocal output with limited recovery time, mirroring vocal changes very similar to those experienced and reported over decades by educators.

Voice care

Earlier in this chapter, aspects of training provision were highlighted, as was the increased concern shown by the European Union for issues of occupational health. Although this attention is welcome, it would also be encouraging to note more direct involvement by the teaching profession to give voice care and development a higher priority.

Alongside the wastage to the profession from those whose voice problems prevent them from continuing in their professional role should be set the many hundreds of hours lost through laryngitis, episodic voice loss and vocal misuse experienced annually by teachers. If, as reported by Verdolini and Ramig (2001), a quarter of the US workforce experiences daily voice problems, then a UK estimate based on the US figures would suggest over 5 million workers are routinely affected by voice loss in the UK, at an annual cost of over £200 million (Hazards, 2004). In the UK, the Health and Safety Executive (HSE) has no figures on the extent of occupational voice loss. However, the vulnerability of teachers, lecturers and trainers to voice problems has already been discussed. It should also be noted that many in a teaching role never get as far as the speech and language therapy clinic, fearing that self disclosure of a problem, which has the potential to affect or even curtail their ability to teach, could signal professional 'vulnerability'. Considering the already noted lack of importance given to vocal change or voice disorders their fear may indeed be realistic.

When questioned by the authors, educators who have had voice problems reported that when this was brought to the attention of the school there had been support from the relevant authorities. Newly qualified teachers reported that they received considerable support from experienced teachers during their probationary and early teaching period. Anecdotal evidence, however, suggests that many teachers arrange therapy sessions out of school hours; some indeed never mention the fact that they are undergoing therapy to colleagues or pupils. For those teachers, lecturers and trainers who do not seek help, their only recourse is to try to continue to teach through periods of laryngitis or voice loss – until the next time. Where voice therapy is not provided as part of a free National Health scheme (as it is in the UK), those with medical insurance may well find treatment costs are covered. For others, the extent of treatment required and the cost of said treatment may be insupportable.

In the UK, information regarding vocal health is available from organizations such as The British Voice Association and the Five Main Voices for Effective Training. Different countries will offer locally specific training through preventive training courses and workshops. Many interdisciplinary voice clinics in the UK offer treatment from a laryngologist, a speech and language therapist, and sometimes, an osteopath, an Alexander Technique teacher, and an experienced, trained singing teacher.

While it is most important to encourage the school or college to invite 'voice' professionals in to offer voice care advice to the staff, it is also recommended that advice is sought from Occupational Health professionals to note elements that are 'hazardous' to good voice use, such as difficult acoustic spaces, lack of hydration and ambient noise levels. Overriding this external advice, however, is the need for individual teachers, lecturers and trainers to take responsibility for their own health.

The Checklists and Voice Performance Review provided on the following pages offer suggestions as to ways in which individuals can monitor and take personal responsibility for reducing external factors in their work environment that may compromise their own voices. They may also be shared with colleagues who may be experiencing similar vocal symptoms and concerns.

- The Occupational Environmental Checklist (Checklist 1.1) offers a way by which to monitor aspects such as air circulation, hydration, dust, heat and noise levels within the classroom.
- The Occupational Vocal Demand Checklist (Checklist 1.2) offers a way by which to monitor work based vocal demands in relation to your own voice.
- The Occupational Vocal Care Checklist (Checklist 1.3) offers a way by which to monitor and check your own voice use periodically.
- The Occupational Acoustic Checklist (Checklist 1.4) offers a way in which to assess the acoustics within the classroom.
- The Voice Performance Review offers a way by which to monitor vocal, emotional and physical change in relation to your own voice over specific time periods.

All of these separate yet interdependent aspects of vocal health, vocal care, vocal demand, vocal performance, acoustic influence on voice and environmental features will be fully dealt with in the following chapters, in order to mitigate potential vocal misuse and highlight ways in which the teaching voice can be maintained throughout a professional career in education.

Checklist 1.1: The Occupational Environmental Checklist

	Yes	No
Are you in a dry atmosphere for a large part of the working day?		
Are you able to alter the room temperature level at work?		
Do you work in a room with poor air quality for long periods of time?		
Does your journey to and from work involve periods exposed to traffic fumes or poorly circulating air?		
Do you work in different physical spaces during the day? For example, do you move from indoors to outdoors?		
Do you work in a difficult acoustic environment?		
Do you feel you have sufficient voice rest periods during your working day?		
Would vocal strain be reduced by adaptations to your workplace?		
Do you remain sitting or standing in one position for long periods of time while at work?		
Do your experience any physical discomfort such as back pain, stiff neck or shoulders as a result of your work?		

Checklist 1.2: The Occupational Vocal Demand Checklist

	Yes	No
Do you use your voice a lot at work?		
Do you have to speak for long periods at work without rest?		
Do you have to speak over background noise, e.g. groups of people or musical or mechanical equipment when at work?		
Could you continue in your current employment if you 'lost' your voice?		
Have you ever had to change your job because of a voice problem?		
Do you regularly work with anyone who has a hearing loss?		
Do you put too many demands on your voice at work?		
Do you feel that the more you use your voice the worse the vocal quality becomes?		
Do you notice an improvement in your vocal quality with rest?		
Do you feel your vocal quality is better after time away from work?		

Checklist 1.3: The Occupational Vocal Care Checklist

	Yes	No
Do you smoke?		
Do you drink a lot of tea, coffee or other drinks containing caffeine?		
Do you drink water throughout the day at work?		
Do you frequently eat dairy produce and/or carbohydrates?		
Do you have irregular meal times?		
Do you experience reflux on a regular basis?		
Do you often shout?		
Do you feel you neglect to care for your voice?		
Do you ever worry about your voice?		
Are you ever hoarse after a night out?		
Do you use an inhaler for preventing or relieving an asthma attack?		
If you answered 'yes', do you use a spacer when using your inhaler?		

Checklist 1.4: The Occupational Vocal Care Checklist

	Yes	No
Is your work place situated on or near a busy road, transport hub, or building site?		
Is your work place sited under an airport flight path?		
Is your work place designated as open plan?		
Does your work place meet nationally recognized acoustic building regulations?		
Is the acoustic environment given significance in your work place?		
Has your work place been acoustically assessed in relation to the levels of reverberation in the classroom or lecture theatre?		
Has there been an assessment of the acoustic properties of your work place by a trained acoustician?		
Have you been offered any advice regarding acoustic modification of your work place to militate against vocal disorders?		
Is there an auditory induction loop in your workplace?		
Are there aspects of the room that interfere with easy voice use, e.g., a lot of glass, hard surfaces, very high or low ceilings, carpet?		

The Voice Performance Review

Use this sheet to review how you have been feeling and what, if any, changes you have noticed that affect your voice in a specific time period.

Dates From: To:		
	Yes	No
During this period the quality of my voice has:		
Remained the same		
Remained flexible		
Become increasingly strained		
Become more breathy		
Become increasingly husky		
Become more harsh		
Become lower in pitch		
Become higher in pitch		
Started to 'cut out' while I am speaking		
During this period I have:		
Felt very tired		
Felt quite run down		
Felt not very healthy		
Felt not at all energetic		
Had days off work through illness		

	Yes	No
Remained very fit		
Remained energetic		
Remained very healthy		
During this period I have:		
Felt quite stressed		
Felt generally quite anxious		
Felt depressed		
Felt generally quite angry		
Felt positive		
Felt quite calm		
Felt as though I could cope well at work and at home		
Not noticed any change in my emotional health		
During this period I have:		
Found it easy to make myself heard		
Found it difficult to make myself heard		
Found that sometimes my voice 'fades' away the longer I use it		
Found it difficult to change the volume of my voice		
Found it difficult to change the pitch of my voice		
Found that I have sometimes 'lost' my voice when speaking		

	Yes	No
Found that I could not predict how my voice would sound when starting to speak		
Found that I often need to clear my throat when I am speaking		
Found that if I am speaking even for a short time I begin to cough		

```
Chapter outline

The role of voice in the communication process
Voice care and training provision
Vocal requirements for teaching
Physical challenges of the classroom setting
Classroom noise
Classroom design
Classroom ergonomics
Vocal awareness
Additional vocal challenges
Voice care
Occupational Environmental Checklist
Occupational Vocal Demand Checklist
Occupational Vocal Care Checklist
Occupational Acoustic Checklist
The Voice Performance Review
```

References and further reading

Angelillo M, DiMaaio G, Costa G, *et al.* 2009. Prevalence of occupational voice disorders in teachers. *Journal of Preventive Medicine and Hygiene* **50**: 26–32.

Bowers T and McIver M. 2000. Ill health retirement and absenteeism mongst teachers. Cambridge: Department for Education and Employment. Available at: <http://dera. ioe.ac.uk/4471/1/RR235.pdf> [Accessed August 2017].

De Jong FICRS, Kooijman PGC, Thomas G, Huinck WJ, Graamans K, Schutte HK, *et al.* 2006. Epidemiology of voice problems in Dutch teachers. *Folia Phoniatrica et Logopaedica* **58**: 186–98.

Department for Education. *Get into Teaching*. Available at: <https://getintoteaching.education.gov.uk/explore-my-options/teacher-training-routes> [Accessed August 2017].

Dickson DA, Hargie ODW, and Morrow NC. 1989. *Communication Skills Training For Health Professionals: An instructor's handbook*. London: Chapman and Hall.

Greenland EE and Shield BM. 2011. A survey of acoustic conditions in semi-open plan classrooms in the United Kingdom. *The Journal of the Acoustical Society of America* **130**(3): 1399.

Government Equalities Office. 2010. *Disability Discrimination Act 2010.* Available at: <https://www.gov.uk/guidance/equality-act-2010-guidance> [Accessed August 2017].

Government Equalities Office. 2010. *Equality Act 2010* [On 1 October 2010, the Disability Discrimination Act became part of the Equality Act 2010 (EqA)]. < https://www.gov.uk/guidance/equality-act-2010-guidance> [Accessed August 2017].

Hargie O (ed). 2006. *The Handbook of Communication Skills.* London and New York, NY: Routledge.

Hazards Magazine. 2010. Teacher gets voice loss payouts but will never teach again. Issue 112: October–December. Available at: <http://www.hazards.org/voiceloss/voicelessons.htm> [Accessed August 2017].

Hazards Magazine. 2004. Work Hoarse. Issue 88: October–December. Available at: <http://www.hazards.org/voiceloss/workhoarse.htm> [Accessed August 2017].

Health and Safety Executive. 1974. *Health and Safety at Work Act 1974.* Available at: <http://ww.hse.gov.uk/legislation/hswa.htm> [Accessed August 2017].

Hendy L and Parke S. 2015 *Five Main Voices for Effective Training.* Available at: <http://www.the5voices.com/> [Accessed August 2017].

HM Government. 2015. *The Building Regulations &c. (Amendment) Regulations 2015,* No 767. Available at: <http://www.legislation.gov.uk/uksi/2015/767/contents/made> [Accessed August 2017].

Hume SB and Wegman A. 2016. Preventing vocal burnout in future teachers. Poster presentation at *ASHA Convention 2016.* Available at: http://blog.talktools.com/wp-content/uploads/2016/11/Hume-Wegmans-2016-ASHA-Poster.pdf [Accessed August 2017].

Industrial Injuries Advisory Council. 2006. Available at: <http://www.iiac.org.uk> [Accessed August 2017].

Hunter EJ, Titze IR. 2010. Variations in intensity, fundamental frequency and voicing for teachers in occupational versus non occupational settings. *Journal of Speech, Language, Hearing Research* **53**: 862–75.

Investopedia. 2013. The causes and costs of absenteeism in the workplace. *Forbes Magazine,* 10 July. Available at: <http://www.forbes.com/sites/investopedia/2013/07/10/

the-causes-and-costs-of-absenteeism-in-the-workplace/#27221c43bd30> [Accessed August 2017].

Hunter EJ and Titze IR. 2010. Variations in intensity, fundamental frequency and voicing for teachers in occupational versus non occupational settings. *Journal of Speech, Language, Hearing Research* **53**: 862–75.

Koufman JA. *What are Voice Disorders and Who Gets Them?* Available at: <http://www.speechpathology.com/articles/what-voice-disorders-and-who-1508-1508> [Accessed August 2017].

Lemov D. 2010. *Teach like a Champion.* San Francisco, CA: Jossey-Bass, Wiley Imprint.

Lockhart M. 2008. *The Breathing and Voice Workout.* Unpublished exercise programme.

Martin S. 2003. An exploration of factors which have an impact on the vocal performance and vocal effectiveness of newly qualified teachers/lecturers. PhD thesis, University of Greenwich.

Mattiske JA, Oates MJ, and Greenwood KM. 1998. Vocal problems among teachers: a review of prevalence, causes, prevention, and treatment. *Journal of Voice* **12**: 489–99.

McSporran E. 1997. Towards better listening and learning in the classroom. *Educational Review* **49**: 102–11.

Morton V and Watson DR. 1998. The teaching voice: problems and perceptions. *Logopedics Phoniatrics Vocology* **23**: 133–9.

Morton V and Watson DR. 2001. The impact of impaired vocal quality on children's ability to process spoken language. *Logopedics Phoniatrics Vocology* **26**(1): 17–25.

Nerrière E, Vercambre M-N, Gilbert F, and Kovess-Masféty V. 2009. Voice disorders and mental health in teachers: a cross-sectional nationwide study. *BMC Public Health* **9**: 370. <Available at: <https://www.ncbi.nlm.nih.gov/pmc/articles/PMC2762990/> [Accessed August 2017].

Ofqual. 2015. *GCSE Reform: Regulations for English language.* Available at: <www.gov.uk/government/consultations/gcse-reform-regulations-for-english-language> [Accessed August 2017].

Ohlsson A-C, Andersson EM, Södersten M, *et al.* 2016 Voice disorders and mental health in teachers: a cross-sectional nationwide study. *Journal of Voice* **30**(6): 755.e13–755.e24 doi:10.1016/j.jvoice.2015.09.004.

Ohlsson AC, Andersson EM, Sodersten M, *et al*. 2012. Prevalence of voice symptoms and risk factor in teacher students. *Journal of Voice* 26(5): 629–34.

Oldfield P. 1995. *PAT Fact Sheet* (Professional Association of Teachers).

Preciado-Lopez J, Perez-Fernandezz C, Calzada-Uriondo M, and Preciado-Ruiz P. 2008. Epidemiological study of voice disorders among teaching professionals of La Rioja, Spain. *Journal of Voice* 22(4): 489–508.

Roche F. 2016. *State of Education Survey Report*. The Key. Available at: <https://view.joomag. com/state-of-education-report-2017/0676372001494577623> [Accessed August 2107].

Rogerson J and Dodd B. 2005. Is there an effect of dysphonic teachers' voices on children's processing of spoken language? *Journal of Voice* 19(1): 47–60.

Roy N, Merrill RM, Thibeault S, and Smith EM. 2004. Voice disorders in teachers and the general population: effects on work performance, attendance and future career choices. *Journal of Speech, Language and Hearing Research* 47: 542–51.

Roy N, Merill RM, Thibeault S, *et al*. 2004 Prevalence of voice disorders in teachers and general population. *Journal of Voice* 47: 281–93.

Schneider E. 2005. *Noise in Figures*. Luxembourg: European Agency for Safety and Health at Work. Available at: <https://osha.europa.eu/en/tools-and-publications/publications/ reports/6905723> [Accessed August 2017].

Shannon C and Weaver W. 1949. *The Mathematical Theory of Communication*. Urbana and Chicago, IL: University of Illinois Press.

Shield BM, Conetta R, Dockerell J, *et al*. 2015. A survey of acoustic conditions and noise levels in secondary school classrooms in England. *Journal of the Acoustical Society of America* 137(1): 177–88.

TeachFirst. Available at: <https://www.teachfirst.org.uk/> [Accessed August 2017].

TeachFirst (Graduates). Available at: <https://graduates.teachfirst.org.uk/> [Accessed August 2017].

Trinite B. 2017 Epidemiology of voice disorders in Latvian school teachers. *Journal of Voice* 2(4): 508.e1–508.e9. doi:10.1016/j.jvoice.2015.09.004 [Accessed August 2017]

University of Iowa, Voice Academy. *The Numbers Don't Lie*. Available at: <https://uiowa. edu/voice-academy/numbers-dont-lie> [Accessed August 2017].

Verdolini K and Ramig LO. 2001. Review: Occupational risks for voice problems. *Logopedics, Phoniatrics, and Vocology* 26: 37–46.

Vilkman E. 2000. Voice problems at work: A challenge for occupational safety and health arrangement. *Folia Phoniatrica et Logopaedica* **52**: 120–5.

Vilkman E. 2004. Occupational safety and health aspects of voice and speech professions. *Folia Phoniatrica et Logopaedica* **56**: 220–53.

Williams NR. 2003. Occupational groups at risk of voice disorders: a review of the literature. *Occupational Medicine* **53**: 456–60.

WHO. 2001. *Occupational and Community Noise: Fact Sheet 258* (rev. Feb. 2001). Available at: <http://collections.infocollections.org/ukedu/en/d/Js0536e/> [Accessed August 2017].

2

How the voice works

For most people, voice, the process that changes silent thought into spoken word, is something that just 'happens'. You think of something to say, you say it, and how it actually happens is rarely, if ever, thought about until something goes wrong. Even then, the mechanics of voice production, why or how the voice has 'gone wrong' are generally unknown. The most usually cited 'cure-all' is either a hot drink with honey and lemon to 'soothe' the voice, or a period without talking to 'rest' the voice. More often, however, the response is to struggle on with faint cries of 'it will get better by itself, just give it a few days' and often that is exactly what happens. For the educator, voice rest over a weekend or holiday period may well bring about improvement and the voice seems a lot better. The individual heaves a sigh of relief and keeps on using the voice in exactly the same way, until the next time and inevitably there will be a next time.

Misuse of the voice

It is difficult to think of any other injury paid as little attention as a voice injury, either by the individual or those they encounter. In general, if muscle strain, back problems, a broken leg, or a sprained wrist are experienced, an individual will take considerable care to avoid any likelihood of it happening again. With voice disorders, however, there appears to be little, if any, attempt to try to avoid it happening again. Whether this be by ignoring the danger of remaining in a smoky atmosphere, a dusty environment, or in a space with a high noise level, the individual, rather than immediately making a fast exit in order to preserve voice, usually responds by 'sitting tight'. Justification for this comes with the words 'it would seem anti-social if I left', or 'I will probably be fine after a night's sleep', even 'perhaps I will get used to it after a while'. Sore throats and voices that rasp perilously out of control from treble to bass are similarly ignored.

So why does vocal misuse continue to occur? If, for example, a man with a large bruise on his leg was seen using his other leg to bang against it, or to hit his injured arm with his fist, it would undoubtedly be seen as somewhat bizarre behaviour. So what makes the voice so prone to self-inflicted vandalism? Part of the answer must lie in the fact that the damage sustained by the vocal folds cannot be seen and indeed, may not really be felt, so any suggestion that damage is occurring is met with some indifference. The voice that is slightly husky and breathy as a result of injury is often described as 'sexy' rather than damaged or vulnerable. Indeed, a vocal quality that is low in pitch is often preferred to that of an overly high pitch, which can be perceived as shrill and unpleasant to listen to. As a consequence, a 'low' but potentially 'injured' voice can evoke limited comment or concern.

Just as some individuals can run for miles without training and without tiring while others will wilt after the first half-mile, so with the voice. Some individuals are less vocally robust than others; they cannot easily sustain extended periods of voice use as the vocal load is genuinely too great. For that reason it is important to recognize and accept one's vocal limitations and avoid situations that exacerbate problems. A useful analogy is that of driving a car. We avoid hazards on the road ahead and while we may not be able to name each individual component in the engine, we listen to the engine noise, generally recognizing when it 'doesn't sound right'.

Knowledge of the function and structure of the voice (the vocal process) is not a prerequisite for effective occupational voice use, but what is not in question is that professional voice users should be secure in the knowledge that their voices are efficient, effective and reliable. In order to achieve that efficiency, effectiveness and reliability, it is important that vocal hygiene and conservation is promoted and encouraged by considering the following recommendations:

Vocal hygiene and conservation

- Be aware and knowledgeable of one's own voice.
- Understand its strengths and limitations.
- Listen to and monitor vocal quality.
- Be sensitive to vocal change.
- Note vocal strain.
- Predict vocal demands and adjust personal voice use accordingly.
- Seek professional help when necessary.
- Never disregard vocal strain or 'soldier on' when it occurs.
- Recognize and avoid situations that are vocally hazardous.
- Do not inhibit vocal freedom or limit the expressivity of the voice through an over scrupulous regard for what is happening within the larynx as this may create unwanted tension.
- Concern and caution, not fear and stress, should be the motivation for change.

Developing vocal awareness

Through the delivery of more training and increased vocal health education provision, increased vocal awareness can be successfully achieved in order to prepare teachers and lecturers for the demands of the teaching role.

Each one of us has a voice that is unique, one that can be instantly identified as belonging to us, and indeed we could say 'we are our voice'. We can achieve change, in terms of altering the volume, speed and pitch of our voices, while still retaining the unique qualities that identify them as our voices.

The different aspects of voice that will be addressed in this chapter are:

- What is voice?
- Where does it come from?

- What is the process that changes silent thought into spoken word?
- Why should it be of interest to professional voice users?

Readers will have their own preference in terms of learning styles (the way in which they best absorb and understand information), be that by learning through listening, learning by seeing or learning by doing. Accommodating individual learning styles is not possible within the scope of this book, so for those whose preference would be for very detailed information there are many widely available excellent resources both in texts and online, detailing the anatomy, physiology and neuro-anatomy of voice production. For others, a simplified but accessible overview of vocal structure and function will be considered sufficient and it is to those readers that the remainder of this chapter is directed.

The process of producing voice

Voice production is dependent on three different but interrelated systems:

- respiratory – responsible for the manner and pattern of breathing;
- phonatory – responsible for how sound is produced at the level of the larynx; and
- resonatory - responsible for modification of this sound.

These separate but interconnecting systems have been adapted to work together in the process of voice production, and are examined below in more detail.

The respiratory system

The main purpose of the respiratory system is to maintain life by carrying air into the lungs where the exchange of the gases oxygen and carbon dioxide takes place. The respiratory system begins at the nose and mouth and ends with the alveoli in the lungs.

The upper respiratory tract consists of:

- the nasal and oral cavities (the nose and the mouth, respectively); and
- the pharynx and larynx.

In addition to its role in respiration, the upper respiratory tract functions in the processes of swallowing, chewing, articulation, resonance and phonation.

The lower respiratory tract consists of:

- the trachea;
- the bronchi; and
- the lungs (housed within the bony thoracic or chest cavity).

Unlike the upper respiratory tract, the lower respiratory tract functions exclusively for the processes of breathing for life support and for the production of speech.

The respiratory tract has two parallel entrances, the nose and the mouth, through which air enters. These merge into a common tract or pharynx. The area within the pharynx immediately behind the nose (called the nasopharynx) and the area behind the mouth (called the oropharynx) are separated by the soft palate, a muscular valve which, when raised, can close off one section from another so that when we swallow, food and liquid do not escape through the nose. In the production of nasal consonants /n/, /m/, and /ng/ the soft palate is lowered to allow these sounds to be resonated in the nose.

Passing through the larynx and the open vocal folds, the respiratory tract continues into the trachea. This divides into two branches then subsequently into the smaller bronchi which enter the lungs and ultimately, into the even smaller alveoli.

The lungs are encased by the bony thoracic skeleton or ribcage, consisting of 12 pairs of ribs. Each set of ribs has different dimensions and degrees of flexibility of movement:

- The first pair of ribs is the shortest and is immobile, fused at the front to the sternum or breastbone and at the back to the spinal vertebrae.
- Pairs two to seven are similarly attached but by synovial joints which permit a degree of rotation.

- Pairs eight to 10 are attached to each other at the front by flexible cartilage.
- Pairs 11 and 12 (sometimes referred to as 'floating ribs') are fixed at the back to the spinal vertebrae but have no fixed attachment at the front.

The arrangement of the ribs is important because the lungs are contained within this bony cage and linked to it by pleural and membranous tissue. The greater the expansion of the thoracic cavity, the greater the volume of air that can be contained within the lungs and, in order to achieve this, the individual must rely on muscular flexibility and support. It is therefore essential that the respiratory muscles are as flexible and efficient as possible in order to achieve this movement of the ribcage.

The orientation of the ribs controls their mobility and this flexible cavity, which also contains major organs such as the heart, the aorta and the vena cava, the trachea and oesophagus, can then accommodate changes in the size of the pear-shaped lungs to contain greater amounts of air needed to support speech or song. The expansion is limited to the base of the lungs because the tops of the lungs are constrained by the fixed immobile ribs at the top of the ribcage. For passive respiration, the movement is so limited that these changes are rarely noticed; it is only when additional air is taken in to support speech or song that the increased movement of the ribcage may be readily identified.

There is a difference between quiet, passive, at-rest 'breathing for life', during which equal phases of breathing in and breathing out occur, and that for the purposes of speech and song where the cycle is modified to allow a quick intake and slow release of air. This slow release of air requires much more active muscular control of breathing than that for breathing for life. Muscular control of breathing requires the active use of several muscles whose effectiveness in supporting breath is very much affected by posture and tension (see box opposite).

Muscles of inspiration (used when breathing in)

Responsible for raising the ribcage and increasing the thoracic volume:

- The diaphragm: this large dome-shaped involuntary muscle is of great importance in breathing, playing the chief part in filling the lungs. During sleep and unconsciousness it maintains respiration under involuntary control.
- External intercostal muscles act to control the amount of space between the ribs and help air intake.
- Accessory neck muscles act to help to raise the first and second ribs when breathing in.
- Accessory back muscles contribute to rib movement when breathing in.
- Accessory pectoral muscles contribute to expansion of the upper ribcage.

Muscles of expiration (used when breathing out)

Responsible for lowering the ribcage and decreasing the thoracic volume:

- Abdominal muscles: responsible for a decrease in the dimensions of the thoracic cavity, helping air to flow out of the lungs.
- Back muscles act in aiding the ribs to depress.
- Internal intercostal muscles act to help control the amount of space between the ribs.

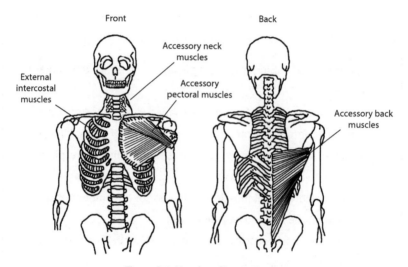

Figure 2.1: Muscles of inspiration.

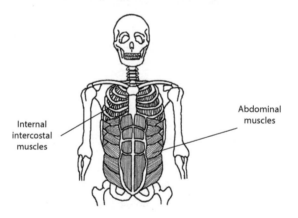

Figure 2.2: Muscles of expiration.

When looking at the figures (Figure 2.1: Muscles of inspiration and Figure 2.2: Muscles of expiration) it is clear that habitual poor posture will make it difficult to achieve optimum breath support. As a consequence the vocal folds (often referred to as vocal cords) will have much less support in terms of initiating and sustaining phonation. High shoulder posture, back and neck tension will all affect smooth muscle movement. A critical first step in achieving easier voicing is through relaxation exercises. Suggestions for general and specific relaxation exercises have been included in Chapter 11.

The phonatory system

This system produces the sounds that the listener translates into speech or song. It consists of the larynx or, as it is often heard referred to, 'the voice box', its muscles and ligaments, and the hyoid bone, which although not actually part of the larynx has an important role as many of the extrinsic muscles of the larynx have an attachment to it. Continuous with the trachea below and the pharynx above, the principal biological function of the larynx is to act as a valve. This valve prevents air from escaping from the lungs, prevents foreign substances from entering the larynx and expels those foreign substances that bypass the epiglottis and threaten to enter the trachea. The valving action of the vocal folds increases intra-thoracic pressure which helps when weight bearing, lifting, coughing, defecation and childbirth.

Energy, in the form of air from the lungs, passes into the trachea and the larynx. The larynx is the principal structure for producing a vibrating air-stream and the vocal folds, which are part of the larynx, make up the vibrating elements.

The larynx is:

- approximately 5 cm long, much smaller in size than might be expected;
- situated in the neck at the level of the third to sixth cervical verte-brae, extending from the base of the tongue to the trachea; and
- made up of nine individual cartilages:
  - three large single cartilages: the thyroid, cricoid, and epiglottis, and
  - three paired cartilages: the arytenoid, corniculate, and cuneiform.

The principal cartilages of the larynx are:

- **The epiglottis.** A broad leaf-shaped cartilage, which is attached to the thyroid cartilage and projects upwards towards the tongue. The epiglottis changes position with tongue movements and alters the size and shape of the pharyngeal cavity.

- **The thyroid cartilage.** The biggest cartilage is shaped like a shield and forms most of the front and side walls of the larynx. It is composed of four quadrilateral plates fused at the front, and this junction or angle of the thyroid is most visible in men and commonly called the 'Adam's apple'. The vocal folds extend from the inside of the thyroid angle to the arytenoid cartilages.
- **The cricoid cartilage.** Forming the base of the larynx, and sitting just below the thyroid cartilage and immediately above the trachea, it is attached to the thyroid cartilage by the cricotracheal ligament. In shape it is broad and flat at the back and narrow at the front.
- **The arytenoid cartilage.** Small pyramid-shaped cartilages which articulate with the cricoid cartilage via the cricoarytenoid joints. The arytenoids are the vocal gymnasts; they can glide medially and laterally and rotate slightly, and may also slide forwards and backwards but with restricted movement. Almost any combination of the above can occur simultaneously. Their importance in the production of voice lies in the fact that the vocal folds have an attachment to these cartilages via the vocal process, so that the specialized nature of their movements is essential in allowing the vocal folds to open and close with ease and thus produce changes in pitch.

Figure 2.4 is a schematic illustration of the movement of the arytenoid cartilages showing the movement of the vocal folds (vocal cords): (a) closing and (b) opening.

The vocal folds

The vocal folds are long, smoothly rounded bands of muscle tissue which may be lengthened, shortened, tensed, and relaxed, as well as opened and closed across the airway. A fuller description of the vocal folds is offered below.

The paired thyroarytenoid muscles make up the body of the vocal fold. The vocal folds consist of:

- the outer layer which maintains the shape of the vocal fold;
- the middle layer comprising three layers of connective tissue; and

42

- the body or vocalis muscle which can thicken, shorten, and stiffen the vocal folds.

The very specialized structure of the vocal folds, composed of several tissue layers of different thickness and each exhibiting varying mechanical properties important for vibration, allows them to change shape and vibrate at differing speeds and at different points along their length, accounting for the amazing range and versatility of the voice.

The vocal folds are white in colour and, in men, between 17 mm and 23 mm in length; those of women are slightly shorter at approximately 12–17 mm. The larynx is well supplied with mucous glands, thereby lubricating the vocal folds and protecting them in part from the effects of friction. Within the

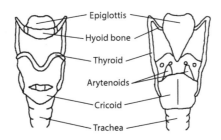

Figure 2.3: Cartilages of the larynx.

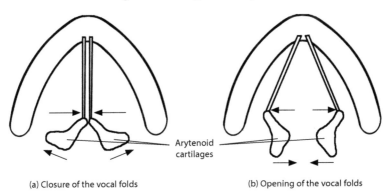

(a) Closure of the vocal folds   (b) Opening of the vocal folds

Figure 2.4: Schematic illustration of the movement of the arytenoid cartilages and consequent movement of the vocal chords.

larynx and the vocal tract the mucous membrane is usually moist, but dryness of the membranous cover of the vocal folds, caused by infection, smoke, and the physiological effects of stress, will noticeably affect the voice.

While the anatomy and physiology of the larynx is well documented, research is ongoing and as more information is gained, so there may be changes as to what is known of the anatomy and physiology of the larynx. It is also important to recognize that individual differences and variability will occur from one larynx to another.

During normal breathing the vocal folds are wide apart, the airstream is unimpeded, and air flows in and out of the lungs in regular phases. For speech, however, the vocal folds are closed or adducted to restrict the flow of air from the lungs, while at the same time air pressure below the folds increases and the vocal folds are literally blown apart, releasing a puff of air into the vocal tract. This release of air results in a decrease in pressure below the folds and the elasticity of the tissue, plus the reduction of air pressure allows them to snap back into their closed position ready to begin this cycle of vocal fold vibration again.

In normal vowel production such vibrations occur at a rate of about 135 complete vibrations per second for men, about 235 vibrations per second for women, and even more for children. This periodic interrupting of the airstream produces a vocal tone that is amplified within the pharyngeal, oral and nasal cavities and transformed through articulation of the lips, tongue, and teeth, resulting in meaningful speech sounds.

The resonatory system

The resonatory system modifies and amplifies the fundamental note and consists of:

- the chest; and
- the pharyngeal, oral, and nasal cavities.

The resonators above the larynx can alter in size, shape, and tension through movement of the base of the tongue and the soft palate. In addition, further modification can occur through contraction of the pharyngeal and extrinsic laryngeal muscles.

Although the larynx is obviously the primary contributor to the production of voice, without the acoustic influence of the resonators the voice would sound very thin indeed. Most of the quality and loudness characteristics associated with the voice are the result of the resonators. In the same way that the weak vibrations of the strings of a musical instrument are altered by the resonating body of the instrument, so the tone that is produced at the level of the larynx, the laryngeal buzz, is altered by the resonators. The airway above the larynx acts like an acoustic filter, which can suppress or maximize some sounds as they pass through. Alterations can also occur in the configuration of the vocal tract by varying tongue positions, raising, or lowering the soft palate, and as an effect of the degree of relaxation or tension present.

The mouth or oral resonator, being the resonator capable of most flexibility of size and shape, is able to enhance natural resonance by producing optimal shapes and so reinforce vibration. Additional resonance can be developed through vowels and voiced nasal consonants /m/, /n/, and /ng/ that add nasal resonance.

For the skilled professional voice user, effective use of the resonators can be a powerful tool in increasing the range, power, and tonality of the voice. A number of exercises to encourage more effective use of the resonators can be found in **Chapter 11**.

Posture and alignment

Voice, as noted above, is the result of a combined effort by all three of the systems, respiratory, phonatory, and resonatory. What must be remembered, however, is that these systems are directly affected by posture. In turn, posture is affected by the movement of the bony skeleton and the muscles and tendons that support the skeleton. Virtually every bone in the body forms a joint, or is connected to some other bone through bone/muscle connection. Muscle is tissue that can contract and relax to cause movement with each muscle attached to two bones, and the push and pull of the muscle moves the bones in

45

relationship to each other. Most muscles are attached to bones by connecting tendons that firmly attach to both the muscle and the bone, connecting the two. Tendons are strong enough to withstand tension when muscles contract to move the bone, although a few muscles attach directly to the bone without a connecting tendon. Ligaments are like tendons made up of strong, fibrous, elastic connective tissue which connects bones to each other in a joint.

This intimate connection allows freedom of movement, but it also means that movement of one body part will affect another either directly or indirectly. The interrelationship of head, neck, and back, and what happens to the positioning of the spine and pelvis, will affect the ribcage and consequently, respiration and voicing. For this reason, when we think of voice work the influence of the whole body needs to be considered, approaching voice holistically rather than attending to the sound in isolation.

The head is balanced on the top of a flexible bony column, the spine, which gives support to the trunk of the body. The spine is made up of 24 small bones called vertebrae; the top seven in the neck are called cervical vertebrae and it is the first of these, the atlas, which supports the skull. Below the neck are the 12 thoracic vertebrae (to which the ribs are attached) and five lumbar vertebrae. Discs of cartilage separate the ring-shaped vertebrae. At the lower end of the spine is the pelvis, the bony structure that connects the spine with the legs, consisting of the hip bones on each side and the sacrum and coccyx behind. The bones of the pelvis protect the soft abdominal organs within them and of course, support the base of the spine. The interrelationship of head, spine, pelvis, and ribcage is, as has been said, critically important for efficient and effective voicing to occur.

Sustained speech and clear vocal quality, imperative for the professional needs of the educator, require good breath support, plenty of air and flexible and relaxed respiratory muscles as well as healthy and flexible vocal folds and uninhibited use of the resonators. Exercises for posture can be found in Chapters 5 and 11.

The ageing process

Changes in vocal quality as a feature of ageing may occur for a variety of reasons throughout adulthood. In some cases these are gender specific, for example, as a result of female hormonal change at puberty, during pregnancy and pre-, during and post-menopause. Temporary changes (except at the menopause) may be the result of a number of factors such as a decrease in oestrogen, water retention, swelling/oedema, dilation of the blood supply to the vocal folds tissue, and increased vocal fold mass.

Hormonal changes account for the voice breaks and uncertain pitch that occur in the male voice at puberty, where the vocal folds increase in length and thickness. For women, hormonal changes at puberty, during menstruation, and during pregnancy cause an increase in fluid retention, resulting in an increase in vocal fold mass, or 'swelling' of the vocal folds. This, in turn, leads to a temporary lowering of the fundamental frequency of the speaking voice, with a subsequent change in vocal quality. Female educators who are using their voices extensively with heavy vocal loading should be particularly aware that their voices might be vulnerable at these times.

The menopause signals a reduction in ovarian hormones and this decrease in oestrogen levels again leads to an increase in vocal fold mass, although instead of this effecting a temporary change in pitch, as in the pre-menstrual period, the change in post-menopausal pitch is permanent. In addition to perceptual voice quality changes such as reduction in pitch and a narrow register (the range of the voice from high to low), other changes occur such as:

- lack of vocal intensity;
- vocal fatigue;
- decreased lubrication of the vocal folds;
- increased rigidity;
- decreased flexibility; and
- rigidity of the cricothryoid muscle.

(NB: the cricothryoid muscle is the only tensor muscle of the larynx to aid phonation; its action tilts the thyroid forward to help tense the vocal folds.)

For some women, however, androgens – which contribute to a loss of secretion – become oestrogen in fat cells, thereby indirectly reversing some of the vocal effects of post-menopausal loss of oestrogen in those women with greater stores of fat cells. It should also be remembered that female hormonal changes do not occur in isolation; significant age-related changes will be occurring throughout the body at the same time, and the effect of these changes on voice quality should not be underestimated.

As with any musical instrument, if the free edges of the vocal folds are damaged, swollen, dry or lacking in tension, the resultant sound will be less than adequate. Typically, swollen vocal folds will give a husky, harsh, breathy quality; the free edges do not meet cleanly to vibrate easily together as a result of the increased mass or swelling, and often air escapes leading to the breathy sound. It should, however, be noted that in many cases the changes are very subtle and may only be perceived by an experienced voice professional.

Changes in pitch level and pitch range in boys' voices, which accompany pubertal change, are well recognized. Hirano *et al.* (1986) suggest that by the age of 15 full vocal ligaments have been developed by both males and females, but the female larynx shows much less dramatic change at puberty than that of the male. For some children, vocal change at puberty can cause considerable emotional trauma. For children who have sung in choirs, either as part of the school curriculum or indeed as a chorister, and have received much praise and recognition for their superb pre-pubertal vocal sound, moving into puberty with much less notable vocal quality can be difficult to come to terms with. Indeed, for many that is the time that they leave choirs as they are uncertain of their vocal output and many never return to singing.

For some young men, despite normal laryngeal growth and the development of secondary sexual characteristics, the new adult male pitch fails to emerge and they retain their pre-pubertal voice. For those young men unhappy with their vocal quality, referral to a speech and language therapist or speech pathologist is available.

Changes in pitch range are also noted as individuals enter 'middle' age. Again differences between male and female voices are noted, specifically at the age at which these changes occur. Ageing changes in the male larynx tend to occur in the fourth decade; for women, as has already been noted, these changes occur at the time of the menopause, usually in the fifth decade. These changes are the result of specific tissue structural changes that occur within the folds:

- The cover undergoes alteration.
- Epithelial thickening is observed (i.e. changes occur in the upper cellular layer of the vocal fold).
- Changes in the underlying connective tissue result in looser linkage of the epithelium to the deeper tissues.
- The elastic fibres of the vocal ligaments break down and become thinner.
- The mucous glands degenerate, resulting in less adequate lubrication of the vocal fold surface.
- Probable changes occur in the biomechanical properties of the superficial epithelium.
- As with other muscles, the laryngeal muscles are prone to atrophy, which means that there are fewer muscle fibres in each muscle.
- In addition, the surviving fibres tend to be thinner and to show significant degenerative changes. It is possible that these changes result from disturbances of the blood supply.

As the vocal folds become less elastic, bowing can occur; the vocal folds do not meet along their full length and consequently, the lack of vibration along their full length leads to a weak breathy note. This seems to be particularly a problem with older men, leading to a thinner higher voice, whereas women, as has been noted, tend to have slightly thicker more swollen vocal folds in older age, limiting their range. In addition there would appear to be a trend towards a decrease in range with increasing age. Laryngeal cartilages calcify, a process that begins quite early in adulthood and starts sooner, and is more complete, in men than in women. The vocal folds of old people look very different from those of younger adults. There is frequently:

- greyish or yellowish discoloration of the tissue;
- loss of mass; and
- a residual gap on vocal fold closure.

There are therefore changes in the sound of the voice and alterations to the larynx that accompany ageing, although it would be inappropriate to suggest that all the changes are the result of alterations to the laryngeal cartilages. Indeed, it may be that the loss of flexibility within the vocal folds means that glottal closure becomes less complete and less stable, and results in a sound that is perceived as being somewhat rough and perhaps breathy. This quality is one that is associated with older individuals.

As well as changes within the larynx, ageing brings about changes within the lungs, which deteriorate with increasing age as noted below. Upper airway disorders may occur with age and sometimes older individuals will develop chronic obstructive pulmonary disease (COPD). Smoking will inevitably accelerate the deterioration of lung function in upper airway disease and indeed may, although not necessarily, have initiated it. Older individuals may also develop late onset asthma in middle to older age. The management of asthma and its effect on the voice is discussed in more detail in **Chapter 3**. Anatomical changes as a result of ageing include:

- a reduction of the mobility of the thoracic cage;
- the ribs becoming less mobile; and
- the lungs and bronchi shrinking and sinking to a lower position in the thorax, although the sensitivity of the airway is reduced and coughing is less likely to occur.

By old age, the vocal changes are quite extensive in both sexes, although they are not inevitable, but certainly vocal deterioration needs to be seen in the light of other changes as a result of ageing such as:

- limited mobility;
- multiple medications;
- lack of motivation or opportunity to communicate;

- reduced hearing; and
- loss of teeth, which causes the upper and lower lips to lose support, and, as a consequence of the loss, the jaw decalcifies and erodes.

Paradoxically, the loss of teeth means the mouth is no longer able to open fully and the joint of the jaw becomes less supple. Mouth opening is of course essential for articulatory precision and for adding oral resonance to the voice. Exercises for increasing and maintaining jaw opening and articulatory muscularity are presented in **Chapter 11**.

Physical activity will prevent noticeable deterioration in respiration, and it is important to avoid pollutants because these will affect the elastic recoil of the lungs. With declining respiratory function, voice quality is affected as a result of lack of breath support. It is likely that changes to the statutory retirement age, which affects pension rights in the UK, will contribute to older individuals remaining in educational roles, so it is important to be aware of vocal change. If, however, attention is paid to postural, respiratory and vocal health, it is possible to maintain a voice that sounds much younger than an individual's chronological age.

Gender identity

For the child who identifies as a different gender, transitioning from male to female (MtF), experiencing a much lower pitch can be very difficult. It is important in terms of the transgendered individual to anticipate likely vocal change, as this may not always be considered and can be of great concern to the individual. Pharmacological solutions, which increasingly are used to suppress pubertal change in pre-pubertal children until advice and counseling have been undertaken, will also serve to suppress pitch change. For individuals who are transitioning at an older age, vocal change will have already taken place. In the case of female to male (FtM) gender change, vocal change is usually managed satisfactorily with the use of hormones to achieve a lower pitch, but in the case of male to female (MtF) gender change, achieving a higher pitch is more difficult. It is not within the scope of this publication to offer therapy intervention, that is for specialist clinicians and multi-disciplinary teams, but exercises for work on pitch given in Chapter 12 offer suggestions which will not infringe professional codes of practice.

Bulimia, anorexia nervosa, substance abuse

Due to their closeness to learners and students, teachers and lecturers are in a privileged position to note voice quality changes that are not due to hormones or puberty but may instead be the result of bulimia or anorexia nervosa. Self-induced vomiting can have a variety of effects on the voice such as:

- hoarseness;
- laryngeal pain;
- voice fatigue;
- phlegm;
- a lower-pitched voice; and
- recurring voice loss.

Educators should be aware of these symptoms as not all those who suffer from bulimia will demonstrate significant weight loss. For those suffering from anorexia, the process of starvation associated with this disorder can affect most organ systems, and the important connection of voice, already noted, to anatomy, physiology, neuro-anatomy, and psychology leads to vocal changes. These may be manifested either in the energy and delivery of voice, or be a result of degenerative changes caused by mineral, bone, or vitamin deficiency. For example, TMJ syndrome, a degenerative arthritis within the tempero-mandibular joint in the jaw (where the lower jaw hinges to the skull), creates pain in the joint area, headaches, and problems chewing and opening/closing the mouth; this will affect speech.

Substance abuse in terms of inhaling drugs such as cocaine or smoking marijuana will also affect vocal quality, often altering the clarity of the note. The heat generated by marijuana will burn the vocal folds, damaging the vocal fold structure. Ingesting cocaine will increase the blood flow to the vocal folds leading to swelling and oedema with consequent change to the vocal quality.

When thinking about vocal quality, the checklists from **Chapter 1** can be used not only to monitor your own voice but that of others. If helpful, share them with others in the staffroom. Think about arranging a staff training evening to discuss voice quality changes that you have noted and any issues of voice care and conservation with other staff members. **Chapter 6** offers institution-wide solutions and strategies that may prove helpful.

Chapter outline

- How the voice works
- Misuse of the voice
- Developing vocal awareness
- The process of producing voice
- The respiratory system
- The phonatory system
- The resonatory system
- Posture and alignment
- The ageing process
- Gender identity
- Bulimia, anorexia, substance abuse

References and further reading

Abitbol J. 2006. *Odyssey of the Voice*. San Diego, CA: Plural Publishing.

Bunch Dayme M. 2005. *The Performer's Voice*. New York, NY and London: WW Norton & Company.

Dacakis G. 2006. Assessment and goals In: Adler RK, Hirsh S, and Mordaunt M (eds), *Voice and Communication Therapy for the Transgender/Transsexual Client*. San Diego, CA: Plural Publishing.

D'haeseleer E, Depypere H, Claeys S, *et al.* 2011. Vocal characteristics of middle-aged pre-menopausal women. *Journal of Voice* 23(3): 360–6.

Hirano M and Kurita S. 1986. Histological structure of the vocal fold and its normal and pathological variation. In: Kirschner JA (ed), *Vocal Fold Histopathology*. Baltimore, MD: College Hill Press.

Martin S and Lockhart M. 2013. *Working with Voice Disorders* (2nd edn). Milton Keynes: Speechmark Publishing Ltd.

Mathieson L. 2001. *Greene and Mathieson's The Voice and its Disorders* (6th edn). Chichester: John Wiley & Sons.

Oates J. 2006. Evidence based practice. In: Adler RK, Hirsh S, and Mordaunt M (eds), *Voice and Communication Therapy for the Transgender/Transsexual Client*. San Diego, CA: Plural Publishing.

3

The effects of extensive vocal use on the voice

Working within the field of occupational voice disorders, and specifically in a training role with educators over many years, the authors were aware of a great many teachers who had previously looked for, with limited success, 'some sort of support group' for their vocal problems; these individuals had been under the (albeit mistaken) impression that they were the only ones suffering from vocal difficulties. They remarked that although colleagues experienced voice loss, this was usually attributed to colds or a virus; no connection was made between extensive voice use or vocal loading and voice loss. A number of educators returned for subsequent training because they felt that not only was additional training needed but also, that contact with the group should be maintained. This served the dual purpose of reassurance and validation: reassurance that they had a legitimate problem and their vocal experiences were common, and validation of their efforts in trying to effect vocal change.

Despite efforts to highlight voice care within education over several decades through the auspices of organizations such as the British Voice Association, the 5 Voices Training Programme, and the former Voice Care Network (organizations which have a long and consistent history of raising the issue of the vocal care of teachers and lecturers), little widespread change has been achieved. The Department for Education (DfE) on their

Healthy Schools Healthy Teachers (2014) website recommends that teachers and trainee teachers should be referred to specialist help from a speech and language therapist and/or an ear, nose and throat (ENT) consultant should they experience vocal problems. A brief reference is to be found in an earlier publication from 2000 entitled 'Fitness to Teach'; this document includes a section with the title 'Occupational Health Guidance for the Training and Employment of Teachers' in which voice trauma is mentioned amongst the physical, chemical and biological hazards noted therein.

Although these initiatives are very much welcomed, vocal health information and vocal care are still not given a high enough priority within education. Paradoxically, one reason for this may be the number of teachers and lecturers in schools or universities who experience voice problems. Studies suggest that between 12 and 25% of educators are affected by voice problems, which in turn, as already noted, may lead to a tacit 'acceptance' of voice problems. An unspoken message of 'this is a problem we all expect to have at some time or another; it will probably improve so don't worry about it' reduces the impact of the problem. Persistent funding difficulties and staff shortages mean that educators are often very reluctant to take time off work with what is perceived as a fairly 'minor' ailment. Indeed, this situation is widespread and underlines the commitment of the majority of those working in education who endeavour to 'keep going', irrespective of the state of their voices. As a result, the serious long term implications of a voice problem may not be seen as demanding particular attention and may, most regrettably, be disregarded. The vocabulary of pain or discomfort is very personal, and educators often find that feelings of vocal discomfort are 'lost in translation' so that the seriousness of the voice disorder may be minimized and as a result, 'early warning' signs of vocal misuse receive a worrying lack of attention.

Gender differences

Much of our early understanding of the complexities of the problems that educators experience came from those individuals who attended In-Service (Inset) training days; we owe a great deal to them. Women far outnumbered men and this reflected a well observed gender difference: men generally experience fewer episodes of voice loss than women, resulting partly from their ability to achieve volume without strain and the greater resonance, and therefore carrying power, of the male voice. Allied to this is a sociological element; despite attempts to eliminate gender bias, the deeper male voice is often perceived as possessing greater authority and gravitas than the lighter female voice. Learners and students may therefore listen more intently and more quietly to the male voice, and thus reduce the number of episodes where the male teacher or lecturer has to shout above class room noise, in turn reducing episodes of vocal misuse. There are of course exceptions to every rule and those men who did attend the workshops often appeared more than usually anxious about their voices and under intense concomitant stress. Rather than perceiving their vocal problems as a symptom of an occupational disorder, many had internalized the problem, seeing it as caused by some shortcoming within themselves. The voice, when used efficiently and effectively, can 'work' for as long as necessary without presenting problems provided that it remains healthy and that the environmental conditions in which it is used are reasonable. Educators often experience vocal loading far in excess of actors, for whom vocal training is a high priority.

Training

As noted in **Chapter 1**, the type of voice training required by an educator is not dissimilar to that required by an actor. The voice is a physical instrument and so training should be given to address:

- posture and alignment;
- efficient use of effort;
- breathing;
- voice production;
- vocal quality;
- projection;
- volume;

- interpretative skills; and
- vocal health.

Exercises in Chapters 10, 11, and 12 target all of the aspects above. Chapter 6 has a specific focus on preventative vocal care, while vocal health is a recurrent theme throughout the book.

The effects of teaching on the voice

When questioned by the authors about the effects of teaching on the voice, educators consistently cited 'vocal tiredness', regardless of whether or not they were encountering vocal problems. Vocal 'tiredness' is neither specific nor easily defined, but it was the initial answer of many teachers. That and their other responses are shown below:

- tiredness;
- hoarseness;
- dryness;
- lack of power;
- inability to communicate effectively;
- lack of flexibility;
- tight and constricted feeling;
- soreness;
- rasping quality;
- monotony;
- voice fading after a few hours; and
- feeling that the voice is 'stuck on one note'.

The authors also asked a group of recently qualified teachers to itemize vocal change since starting to teach, and they identified a similar list of voice quality changes:

- changes in pitch;
- huskiness;
- breathiness;

- harshness;
- vocal strain;
- increased harshness; and
- voice could not operate efficiently over a sustained period of time.

No teacher from either group reported that their voice had strengthened with use during their time in post, which contrasts with the experience of actors who, with the benefit of voice training, often remark that their voice strengthens over the run of a play, generally building in resonance, flexibility, power and range.

Many of the descriptions above refer to changes in vocal quality and vocal endurance. These descriptors indicate changes either to the vocal folds or to the structure and functioning of the larynx; these changes are of considerable concern.

Early warning signs and symptoms

All voice users should be aware of the vocal 'early warning' signs and symptoms noted in the checklist below, and they are urged to refer back to this periodically throughout their careers as a way of monitoring their voice quality and voice use. Educators have indicated anecdotally that there is tendency to ignore such symptoms, ascribing them to tension or stress rather than recognizing that the physical tension they experience often comes from effortful voicing. Feelings of a specific tension site or generalized tension, rather than an inability to produce voice, may well be the first indicator of vocal misuse. It should also be noted that when voicing is effortful, a major contributory factor can be related to habitual posture and muscle state, not just specific tension sites within the vocal tract.

The authors' strong recommendation is not to dismiss vocal change as 'part of the job', but to seek medical advice if experiencing any of the symptoms above for longer than two to three weeks.

Early warning signs and symptoms

	Yes	No
Recurring loss of voice		
Does your voice 'cut out' or do you find it difficult to produce sound for several minutes/hours/days?		
Reduction in both sung or spoken vocal range		
Do you find it difficult (if singing) to reach the high and low notes that you used to produce with ease?		
Do you find that your voice suddenly 'breaks' in the middle of a sentence, going from a higher pitch to a lower pitch or from a whisper back to voice again?		
Reduction in the flexibility of the voice		
Do you find it difficult to use your voice expressively? For example, telling a story or expressing a feeling of joy or sorrow, disinterest, or excitement?		
Pain or discomfort in the area of the larynx		
Does your neck feel uncomfortable?		
Do you ever have a sharp pain in your neck or a feeling of tightness as though your neck was in a vice?		
A feeling of 'tightness/stiffness' in the neck		
Do you feel tension under the jaw particularly in the large tongue muscles, which form a 'strap' under the chin?		

	Yes	No
A marked change in the pitch of the voice after an incident of vocal misuse		
Did you notice your voice changing after shouting, arguing, or after a particular episode of using your voice at high volume?		
A voice that does not return to normal after a cold or a bout of laryngitis		
Did you have a cold or a bout of laryngitis after which you noticed the voice quality was quite changed, perhaps sounding husky or hoarse?		
Loss of volume with an accompanying increase in effort to achieve previous loudness		
Do you notice that you find it difficult and effortful to speak at your normal level of loudness?		
Changes in the free movement of the vocal folds		
Do you notice your voice has a strained quality?		
A feeling of having a 'lump in the throat'		
Do you ever feel as though you have something stuck in your throat all the time, even after swallow--ing, coughing or clearing your throat in an effort to dislodge it? (This is usually a persistent feeling not that experienced when trying to 'swallow one's feelings' in an attempt not to cry).		

	Yes	No
Any loss of hearing		
Do you spend, or have you recently spent, a lot of time with someone with hearing loss? (You may not have noticed that you are speaking with more volume or effort in trying to make yourself understood).		
Have you noticed that your hearing is less acute than it was and if so, can you think about how long it has been since you heard really well? (If hearing loss has been acquired gradually, you may, without realizing it, have been using an increased amount of vocal effort in order to increase the auditory feedback you are getting as a result of reduced hearing).		

Self-monitoring of vocal output

Tension and effortful voicing may also be the result of difficulties in appropriate self-monitoring of the voice. Without training it is very difficult to assess vocal volume levels accurately. The instinctive response when trying to make oneself heard is to increase volume and indeed, at times, shout 'over' noise. Teachers report anecdotally that when a class is making a lot of noise, they try to take control by increasing the effort that they put into producing the sound and endeavour to 'push out' the voice. For untrained voice users this is not only hugely tiring but also counterproductive.

Much of the shouting that occurs in school or college is very damaging to the voice and indeed, very tiring. It is also quite difficult for learners and students, many of whom find constant shouting distracting and at times distressing. In an ideal situation shouting should not be necessary, but even the most resourceful teacher resorts to this very human reaction on occasions. For many teachers, experiencing vocal tension is a daily occurrence; for others this tension, although quite exhausting, does not create permanent vocal problems. For some, however, the legacy of such daily effortful voicing is either vocal damage or a reduction in the range and robustness of the voice.

For most educators, rather than misusing their voices in an attempt to 'shout over' or 'cut through' classroom noise, it is important to acquire skills that conserve the voice by altering their approach to class or group control. As noted earlier, **Chapter 6** looks at personal strategies that may be used in order to care for and preserve the voice, while **Chapter 10** provides detailed exercises and strategies for voice conservation and the safe use of high volume.

Medical referral

Identifying specific muscles or ligaments is difficult for all but the most skilled, so a voice problem arising from muscular tension may, for example, be interpreted as a 'sore' throat. Educators reported anecdotally that they had visited their General Practitioners (GP) to seek help, but, because they were unable to articulate their voice problem clearly, or describe the symptoms with precision, they had left the surgery without the advice and help that they sought.

Within the UK there are considerable demands on GPs and consequent limits on consultation time, so it is entirely possible that voice problems are not always given the attention that they deserve. On occasions, teachers complained that the GP's initial response had often been to write out a prescription. This action, however, often distorts the true significance of the problem for the teacher, whose immediate reaction may be to think 'I'm making a fuss about nothing' or 'It's no wonder my voice is sore, I'm obviously not a good teacher' or 'This is what happens to teachers' voices'.

Teachers report that they consequently feel disinclined to return to the GP, believing that they just have to 'live with it'. Many of the teachers believed that it was not a 'bad enough problem to moan about' in the staff room or to take time off to deal with. A frequently heard comment was:

> Well you can't really take time off for a bad voice, not like you could for tonsillitis; you don't feel ill when your voice is bad.

One teacher said:

> It's not like an ankle; when you sprain your ankle everyone can see you are in trouble and they sympathize. No one can see the voice so they often ignore it.

Another teacher said:

> When my voice is bad, people occasionally say 'you've got a nasty cold'. I don't bother to explain I don't have a cold at all.

It is to be regretted that in the experience of those questioned, few GPs appeared willing to refer teachers to a laryngologist or considered reasons other than viral or bacterial infections as a cause of a voice problem. When attempting to describe the voice problem clearly to the GP it may be useful to think carefully about the aspects in the vocal health inventory below. This will not only allow a more precise description of symptoms, identify possible triggers and trace the progression of the vocal problem but in turn will, it is hoped, help the GP to make a diagnosis. If onward referral to a speech and language therapist/speech pathologist is recommended, the responses to these questions are ones that will be helpful for the GP or speech and language therapist/speech pathologist in reaching a differential diagnosis.

Completion of the personal 'inventory' opposite should allow a clearer picture to emerge of both the onset and the progression of the changes in your vocal quality. In this way certain factors, such as aspects of physical health, mental health or environmental factors, may emerge as being implicated in the voice problem.

Voice diary

Using a voice diary on a weekly basis is a very useful strategy to check the condition/state of your voice over a period of time. The diary allows you to register and quantify periods of: voice rest, easy voicing, vocal stress and vocal loading.

Voice diary			
Week beginning:			
	Morning	Afternoon	Evening
Monday			
Tuesday			
Wednesday			
Thursday			
Friday			
Saturday			
Sunday			

Use a number from the descriptors below to help you make a record of your voice use every day.

1 = voice rest
2 = easy voicing
3 = vocal stress
4 = vocal loading

Vocal health inventory

	Yes	No
Has the voice problem existed for longer than a month?		
Is it related to a cold or flu?		
Do you have asthma?		
Do you regularly use an inhaler?		
Are you ever short of breath?		
Do you regularly have acid reflux?		
Can you remember anything that might have precipitated the voice problem, such as shouting or arguing or talking over loud background noise?		
Does it follow a pattern?		
Is it a recurring problem? For example, do you notice it occurring at the beginning of term or after a half-term or holiday break?		
Is your urine dark in colour instead of pale? Monitor the amount of liquid that you drink each day.		
Have you changed your diet recently?		
Do you have any joint or mobility problems?		
Are you making postural changes in order to accommodate the positioning of the desks or the height of the whiteboard in your workplace?		

	Yes	No
Could your individual teaching style be a contributing factor?		
Do you suffer from backache, neck ache or other physical problems?		
Do you ever get a feeling that you have 'a lump in the throat'?		
Do you feel under professional or personal stress?		
Is there anything you do that helps to reduce the symptoms?		
Are you working in a poor acoustic environment?		

Describing the vocal symptom

As previously stated, the terminology for reporting and defining voice problems is very subjective. Some of the more frequently used 'umbrella terms' are described in more detail below.

Tiredness

Vocal 'tiredness' is usually caused by ineffective production of the voice. The muscles used to produce sound are used in other functions, such as lifting, pushing, giving birth, coughing, and keeping foreign bodies from getting into the lungs. As they possess an innate muscularity they are also capable of being inadvertently over-used in the production of voice. Muscle tension disorders (where there is increased tension in the neck and suprahyoid muscles), with muscle ache and fatigue, are well known effects of vocal misuse. When used efficiently, the voice does not tire. When used without proper breath support and with poorly aligned body posture, or when more muscle effort than necessary is used, the voice begins to tire.

Loss of range and volume

Many educators report that they no longer have the singing range that they used to have, nor can they make themselves heard over 'normal' classroom noise. Indeed, some report that they cannot make themselves heard at the back of the class. Educators who report loss of volume do not always report allied partial or complete voice loss, despite a significant diminution of their vocal range and vocal effectiveness. One of the difficulties of chronic vocal misuse lies in the fact that for many educators, the problem has been slow and insidious. It is only when asked to think back to their vocal function at the beginning of their careers and compare it with their current vocal function that teachers and lecturers appreciate how much their range has diminished. Had the change in voice quality and reduction in vocal range been either more sudden or more complete, then more attention might have been given to the problem, allowing the teacher or lecturer to retain much more vocal flexibility.

Hoarseness/huskiness

In the perceptual description of voice quality the terms 'husky' and 'hoarse' are often combined because they do not stand alone particularly successfully. Associated with breathiness, tension and strain there is generally a rather low, rough (as distinct from breathy) sound. Hoarseness occurs because the vocal folds are swollen and are therefore only partly vibrated along their full length. There is not necessarily any pain or discomfort, although it may be present. The voice in this condition is sometimes described as attractive or even 'sexy' and because of this, individuals may fail to rest the voice to reduce swelling and allow the vocal folds to return to their natural state.

Laryngitis

Vocal symptoms of hoarseness and huskiness may be experienced with laryngitis. In extreme cases the voice may vanish altogether or diminish to a whisper. Educators, as already noted, tend to 'soldier on' ignoring the problem. Disregarding the symptoms is not to be encouraged because when the vocal folds are swollen and closure is incomplete, the muscles of the larynx have to work particularly hard to produce a sound. The volume required to reach the back of the classroom or, worse still, to control a group of noisy children on the sports field results in real strain and can, in severe cases, cause considerable damage to the vocal folds.

Allergies

It is also possible that an allergic reaction may be responsible for a hoarse/ husky vocal quality. This can be related to hayfever or pollution, or allergies such as tree pollen or grass, and can result in either a reduction in the lubrication of the vocal folds or an abundance of mucus. Asthma, with its consequential effect of reducing lung capacity, can contribute to vocal strain and hoarseness. It is often misplaced stoicism that encourages a teacher to continue under these conditions; the voice in this state is seldom effective. The husky voice can have the effect of making an audience feel tired and inattentive. The emotional edge to the voice has gone and the tension that goes into producing the sound becomes the quality that is listened to. It is interesting to observe an audience being addressed by a 'hoarse' speaker; they often clear their throats in sympathy or even cough.

What causes hoarseness?

If there is no cold, bacterial or viral infection, or an allergic condition, there is probably a 'functional' reason for the hoarse sound of the voice. It could be that the individual's posture is not conducive to easy, efficient production of the voice, causing the muscles to overwork and resulting in 'strain'. In an otherwise healthy voice, there is usually a fairly easily correctable reason for the problem that is very often linked to breathing. A fuller description of breathing was given in **Chapter 2** but it is important to reiterate that breath is responsible for the vibration of the folds and, if that breath is either not powerful enough to set the vocal folds in motion or not synchronized with the activity of voice production, problems can occur. Breath is closely linked to our emotional life and so when we are under stress we are more likely to 'block' or inhibit the very natural and spontaneous activity of breathing.

The teacher's perspective

A small-scale, in-depth study conducted by means of a questionnaire (Martin and Darnley, 1996) allowed for an exploration of some of the problems that educators encountered in terms of how their own voices 'performed' under teaching conditions, and how confident or otherwise they were with their own level of language use. The study was conducted in a primary school in a residential area, with no major discipline problems among the children aged from rising 5 to 11 years. A hearing unit attached to the school meant that hearing-impaired learners were integrated into the school. There were children with other special educational needs and disability (SEND) within the school but these represented a small percentage of the school population.

Of the staff who completed the questionnaire:

- 78% had no work on their voice during their training;
- 87% said that their voices had failed at some point in their professional life, becoming croaky, hoarse or husky;
- 21% of those questioned said that their voices had disappeared altogether on occasion;
- 87% said their throats became tight; and
- 65% said that they thought that a feeling of a tight throat was a common complaint.

Despite the difficulties that the staff experienced with their voices, 88% said that it conveyed the qualities that they wanted to convey. However, when asked to describe their voices some of the adjectives used were:

- squeaky;
- quite weak;
- loud;
- husky;
- creaky; and
- low pitched.

Of those questioned, only 22% were happy with their voices as they were.

When asked to name the most difficult vocal situation that they encountered:

- 34% of the teachers named parents' evenings; and
- 23% cited reprimanding the class as the most difficult vocal situation.

The teachers were asked if they saw themselves as performers and all those questioned said 'yes'.

When asked how confident they were with spoken language:

- 65% said that they were confident but, when asked if their confidence would be the same with a different age group, only 22% said 'yes'.

When asked what aspects of teaching they did not feel fully prepared for while training their answers ranged from:

- drama and story-telling;
- the pastoral role of a teacher;
- the stamina required;
- the work levels;
- the amount of talking;
- the use of the voice;
- behaviour management skills.

When asked to elucidate on aspects of concern regarding their vocal health their answers were as follows:

- voice loss;
- changes in vocal quality;
- lack of vocal robustness; and
- anxiety and concern.

Case histories and personal reflections

There is no typical teacher and no typical career pathway, and the transferable skills of educators offer them a wide choice of educational roles. The following case histories are included to offer a personal snapshot of the effect of a voice disorder from the teacher's perspective. They feature aspects of loss of volume, loss of range and complete voice loss. (All names have been changed).

Rosa:

By the 80s, stress had taken its toll and I developed thyroid and stomach ulcer problems which still require medication. At the time I did not relate my voice problems to this. Every couple of years, usually about November time, I would have a short bout of laryngitis which would impact on teaching. Of far greater concern was losing the ability to sing and a 'tickling' incessant cough followed by whispering when I raised my voice or became stressed which continues to date. Some of the ways I tried to adapt were as follows:

- As I was unable to sing anymore, I swapped my singing lessons with another teacher's art lessons by mutual consent and we both benefited – she loved singing and art lessons were usually more peaceful.

- Being the only qualified swimming teacher and lifeguard in the school, I was in charge of swimming lessons but the warm, humid atmosphere and having to use a raised voice due to competition from five other groups teaching at the same time, brought on coughing fits. In the end, groups had to be reorganized and I was left to lifeguard which with hindsight, was probably safer.

- Experiencing a bout of laryngitis whilst trying to take a practical science lesson amidst much noise and excitement, I was unable to make myself heard. As a last resort, I raised my hand in the air. Being a Brown Owl with a local Brownie Pack,

I used the gesture which is used to mean, stop what you are doing, face me and listen. It worked a treat - with the girls! The boys wondered what was going on but were keen to join in once explained. I only used this tactic when nothing else worked in case familiarity bore contempt. Only able to whisper, I used other tactics which focused on pupils doing the lion share of the talking whilst fulfilling targets in the curriculum.

Annie:

Initially, I became a SEND (Special Educational Needs and Disabilities) teacher, but as the years passed by, I was given more and more mainstream English groups to teach, and this is when the vocal difficulties began. I would love to tell you that I was perfect, patient and calm in all my lessons, but sadly I have to admit that I did shout now and then, particularly when teaching Year 9 boys! I also developed adult-onset asthma around this time, which appeared to exacerbate the problem further.

I eventually saw a consultant, who concluded that the inhalers I was prescribed were causing inflammation of the vocal cords. He was very sympathetic, but could offer no remedy, except a recommendation to inhale Friar's Balsam to help reduce the inflammation. Not very helpful.

I soldiered on, and started to use a spacer with my inhalers, but eventually had to return to the same consultant, as my voice was becoming more and more unreliable. On the second visit, he was much less sympathetic; I hoped he might say I had polyps in the larynx that could be removed by surgery so that I could be 'cured'. Instead, he told me that I was the sixth teacher he had seen that day, and the solution would be to give up my job, but he couldn't tell me to do that! Even less helpful.

Rachael:

At 50, the opportunity to take an early retirement redundancy presented itself, and I decided to give up my job, mainly in order to preserve what was left of my voice (and my stress levels). I didn't stop teaching, however, but continued working as a specialist teacher/assessor; this allowed me to work 1:1, or with very small groups, which meant that I no longer needed to project my voice, although I still had to talk!

Last summer I retired, aged 63, but the knock-on effect of the career choice I made at 50 has had a considerable impact on the pension I now receive.

Singing used to be my greatest passion. I sang all the time as a child, performed solos and was even in a folk band whilst at college. The worst part of this sorry tale is that I completely lost my singing voice, and all I can manage now is a croak. If singing in church, I have to drop an octave, but when I should move up into a higher register, there is just a squeak, or no voice at all. I had hoped to join a choir in my retirement, but that is now impossible, which is a cause of great sadness to me.

Although at college we had lectures and assessments in Speech, as I remember, it was all about content. There was never any advice about projecting one's voice, or training in the use of vocal dynamics as an effective classroom tool, which would have been invaluable, particularly for women, whose voices don't carry as well as men's. In my case, as a trained singer and having done quite a bit of acting, I knew how to use the diaphragm to control my voice in order to avoid vocal strain, but this didn't help to prevent voice loss. I still sound very croaky if I have a cold, or if I am stressed or wheezy.

Michael:

During my career, one colleague (female) had to have an operation on her throat after straining her voice in the classroom for several years. Another, a male PE teacher, has suffered hearing loss/damage from teaching for 30+ years in gyms and sports halls, and using whistles in that sort of an echoing environment. Colleagues also reported loss of voice during Ofsted (Office for Standards in Education) inspections, most probably due to the stress.

Personally, I suffer from quite disabling sore throats during winters. I didn't ever expect sympathy, but the prevailing attitude among management was that such a condition was a poor excuse for absence. I know now, as a singer, that my vocal chords (sic) have suffered, following years of professional abuse.

It was only late in my career that I discovered that I was not alone in this. When I did, and by then as a Professional Development Coordinator in the school, I was able to include advice on vocal control within my induction of new colleagues and trainees. This tied in with the importance of vocal projection, something which trainees often had to be advised about, coached in and reminded of.

Maybe because of our training, I always saw vocal proficiency as an important indicator of teaching strength, status and disciplinary standards. I was always surprised to note how many colleagues either would not, or didn't want to, speak to year group assemblies. I'm not sure if this was a lack of confidence or a view that it was not their role to do so, but I grasped the opportunity when it was offered. Perhaps it was my Subsidiary Drama course, perhaps it is just my personality.

Along with the crucial importance of learning pupil names, vocal projection is essential in matters of classroom, and in the secondary environment, corridor control. Sadly, towards the end of my career, I found that younger colleagues either didn't have the ability, self-assurance or acumen to use their voices as a means of control. Without shouting, one must demonstrate through one's voice, who is in control. The student voice is obviously important in learning, but the teacher's voice is essential in directing and controlling conditions for learning.

Kathryn:

When I returned to teaching after a break, I did a fair bit of supply teaching around the local primary schools. Going in as someone new and unknown has its challenges. The children try the supply teacher out to see how far they can go. I would have really appreciated some help with voice control and usage in those days. It is hard to make yourself understood above the babble of 30 odd voices.

On one occasion I was contacted at mid-day and asked if I would go and teach a class of 5-year-olds for the afternoon session. Apparently the supply teacher had completely 'lost her voice' during the morning session – presumably through inappropriate use. I can't remember if I fared any better.

I consider that learning how to project one's voice is an essential part of teacher training. After all, the throat is a delicate organ and the work of the voice is paramount in gaining control in the classroom. To my mind this runs side by side with body language. I believe training should be given in controlling a class and commanding respect. I don't recall it being a part of my training, but it is essential. So many probationary teachers fall by the wayside – such a waste.

Louisa:

It is important to 'save the voice' by letting other people to do the talking. It doesn't have to be the teacher who reads out a piece of prose or poetry, a list of instructions, facts and figures, etc. – let your students do the work. This allows the voice to 'take a rest' and provides a different focus for the class.

My penultimate job was working for a Further Education training provider. I delivered NVQ (National Vocational Qualification) training to young adults including health care assistants. Much of the training related to effective and appropriate communication. In one session I provided the learners with an amusing and well illustrated hand-out and we discussed how best to work with a client who is hearing-impaired.

Making sure the mouth can be seen as the words are enunciated was one thing we agreed upon. As was making sure the light is on the face and (once again) use of facial gesture and hand gesture. These additional 'supports' to the voice can help to reduce the work that it has to do.

My last job was working as an advocate and advocacy trainer. The role involved supporting the client on the phone and in meetings (with police, lawyers, Social Services, council officers, medical services etc.). One had to simply concentrate on getting the client's point of view, preferences, needs and wants across to the audience. This was a useful lesson in focusing on the main thrust of the case. In teaching it needs self-discipline to keep on track and not wander off on tangents. Planning ahead on how to 'wind up' a presentation is essential.

Chapter outline

- Gender differences
- Training
- The effects of teaching on the voice
- Early warning signs and symptoms
- Self-monitoring and vocal output
- Medical referral
- Voice diary
- Describing the vocal symptoms
- The teacher's perspective
- Case histories and personal reflections

References and further reading

Bunch Dayme M. 2005. *The Performer's Voice*. New York, NY and London: WW Norton & Company.

Roy N, Merrill RM, Thibeault S, and Smith EM. 2004. Voice disorders in teachers and the general population: effect on work performance, attendance and future career choices. *Journal of Speech, Language and Hearing Research* **47**: 542–51.

Titze IR. 2007. Voicing and silence in daily and weekly vocalizations of teachers. *Journal of the Acoustical Society of America* **121**(1): 254–9.

4

External stress factors and the effect on the voice

Prevalence of stress

This chapter looks at stress and the physical effect of stress in general terms. It then focuses specifically on the stress experienced within the field of education. The link between voice, stress and tension will be highlighted in order to focus on how the demands of the educational role, with its attendant stress and tension, can affect voice quality, vocal performance and vocal effectiveness, as a result of the changes that stress imposes both directly and indirectly on the vocal mechanism.

Stress can hit anyone in any work place, and recent research shows that work-related stress is global and widespread. In the UK a government agency, the Health and Safety Executive (HSE), recorded figures for 2013/14 of 487,000 people who were off work suffering from stress, depression and anxiety, an increase of 23,000 since its 2011/12 audit. Work-related stress, depression or anxiety is defined as a harmful reaction to undue pressures and demands placed on people at work (Labour Force Survey, 2016). The European Agency for Safety and Health at work reported that over half of the 550 million working days lost annually in the US from absenteeism are stress related, while the American Institute of Stress suggested in an Integra Survey of 2000 that one million workers are absent every day in the US due to stress.

Stress is a symptom of an organizational problem, not an individual weakness, and while it is not confined to particular sectors, jobs or industries, it is known that teaching incurs a high level of stress. Indeed, the prevalence of teacher stress is a worldwide phenomenon, identified three decades ago, when a study (Coates and Thoresen, 1976) suggested that the number of teachers experiencing high levels of perceived stress was as high as 70%.

Such was the concern about the level of stress experienced by teachers within the UK that the National Association of Schoolmasters/Union of Women Teachers (NASUWT) commissioned a comprehensive study of teacher stress almost a quarter of a century ago (Travers and Cooper, 1993). Their findings indicated that teachers, compared with other highly stressed occupational groups, experienced lower job satisfaction and poorer mental health. Teachers were found to be reporting stress-related manifestations that were far higher than the population norms and of other comparable occupational groups. The study discovered the major areas of job dissatisfaction to be the 'inherent pressure of the job', factors of 'management/structure of the school' and 'lack of status and promotion'.

A European survey conducted by the European Agency for Safety and Health at Work in 2010 in 34 countries with 44,000 workers showed that the education sector was one of the most affected sectors, after the health sector, in terms of workers reporting that they hid or suppressed feelings (30%); this can result in psychological strain. Men (21%) were more likely than women (16%) to report having been subjected to adverse social behaviour. A survey of 500 schools in Europe showed that the stress factors in teachers are primarily reported to be workload and role overload, but it is when work conflicts with private life that the teachers' wellbeing is more likely to be negatively affected. School teachers with large class sizes tend to report higher levels of quantitative demands, work–privacy conflict, noise, voice strain and less opportunity to relax.

Estimates for Great Britain from the Labour Force Survey (LFS, 2016) for 2015/16 show:

- The total number of cases of work-related stress, depression or anxiety was 488,000, a prevalence rate of 1,510 per 100,000 workers.
- The number of new cases was 224,000, an incidence rate of 690 per 100,000 workers. The estimated number and rate have remained broadly flat for more than a decade.
- The total number of working days lost due to this condition in 2015/16 was 11.7 million days. This equated to an average of 23.9 days lost per case.
- In 2015/16 stress accounted for 37% of all work-related ill health cases and 45% of all working days lost due to ill health.
- Stress is more prevalent in public service industries, such as education, health and social care, and public administration and defense.
- Occupational bias: jobs that are common across public service industries (such as healthcare workers, teaching, business, media and public service professionals) show higher levels of stress compared with all jobs.
- The main work factors cited by respondents as causing work-related stress, depression, or anxiety (LFS) were workload pressures, including tight deadlines and too much responsibility, and a lack of managerial support.

Looking at gender differences in work-related stress, given the significantly higher percentage of female teachers and lecturers within education (figures for 2015/16 showed that 70% of all full-time teachers in the UK are female; in secondary schools 60% of all full time teachers are female, while 83% of full time teachers in Nursery and Primary schools are female) it is interesting to note that in the three year period from 2013/14 to 2015/16, females had a statistically higher rate of work-related stress than males. The prevalence rate for work-related stress in males was 1,190 cases per 100,000 workers and in females, 1,820 cases per 100,000 workers.

Differences in age categories were also of note. Within male age categories, the higher rates of work-related stress were in the 45–54 years age range.

Within female age categories, the 35–44 year age range reported the greatest level of work-related stress. Within the age range of 25 to 54 years, the prevalence for work-related stress in females was 6,210 per 100,000 workers, in comparison with that in males of 2960 per 100,000 workers.

Labour Force Survey (2016) suggested that the higher rates reported by females is likely to be a product of the proportion of females in the public services and vocational occupations, such as teaching and nursing, as well as cultural differences in attitudes and beliefs between males and females around the subject of stress.

Changes within the education sector in the UK, be it in primary, secondary, or tertiary education, have been frequent and numerous and have contributed substantially to the stress experienced by teachers in the work place (Wu, 1998). It is not within the scope of this book to itemize the changes or comment on the political, demographic, financial and social factors for these changes. It is, however, important to look at educational change in the context of the individual educator working within this environment who is subject to the inherent tensions and stress that accompany change.

Definition of stress

In any discussion of stress it is important to try to define what is understood by the term 'stress', and that in itself presents a problem as tension, strain and pressure are words that may be used synonymously with 'stress'. Stress may be seen paradoxically as both negative and positive. Stress affects everyone but not to the same extent; it can hit anyone at any level and it is not confined to those with, for example, heavy occupational responsibilities. Recent research shows that work-related stress is widespread and is not confined to particular sectors, jobs or industries. Stress is not an illness – it is a state. However, if stress becomes too excessive and prolonged, mental and physical illness may develop. Work-related stress can be a significant cause of illness and is known to be linked with high levels of sickness absence, staff turnover and other issues. Work-related stress develops because a person is unable to cope with the demands being placed on him/her. Well designed, well organized and well managed workplaces are generally good for us, but if there is insufficient attention to the design, organization, and management of the work place, it can result in work-related stress. The UK HSE's formal definition of work-related stress is: 'The adverse reaction people have to excessive pressures or other types of demand placed on them at work.'

There is a difference between pressure and stress. Pressure can be positive and a motivating factor, and it is often essential in a job. It can help individuals to achieve their goals and perform better. When, however, the demands of their work are perceived by an individual as greater than their ability to cope, stress is experienced. Stress occurs as a natural reaction to too much pressure, but it also provides a necessary and essential 'warning' sign of impending danger or that something is wrong.

Stress may therefore be described as a form of interaction between the environmental demands and an individual's ability to meet those demands. Balancing the demands and pressures of the job by utilizing their skills and knowledge allows an individual to cope with the job without experiencing undue pressure.

Factors in stress

Stress affects people in different ways and what one person finds stressful can be normal to another. Each individual has a unique response to stress; stress perceived by one as beneficial and stimulating, inspiring the individual to perform well, may be perceived as too much by another and thus, the ability to perform well will be impaired. For the individual who responds to stress positively, too little stress can in fact reduce effectiveness and leave the individual listless and under-stimulated.

With each new situation a person will decide what the challenge is and whether he/she has the resources to cope. If that person decides he doesn't have the resources, he will begin to feel stressed. According to the UK HSE, how individuals appraise the situation will depend on various factors, including:

- their background and culture;
- their skills and experience;

- their personality;
- their personal circumstances;
- their individual characteristics;
- their health status;
- their ethnicity, culture, gender, age, or disability; and
- other demands both in and outside their work.

Prevalence of teacher stress

Given that work stress has reached a critical level, and in recognition of the effect of stress on the voice, it is important to examine the prevalence of stress among the teaching profession. In addition, it is vital to acknowledge the extent to which a teacher's working environment contributes to teacher stress.

As long ago as 1999 the Department of Health reported stress at work reaching epidemic proportions (Milne, 1999). It was recognized as the biggest occupational health problem, with up to 6 million working days lost a year at a cost of about £5 billion.

There is little to suggest that anything has changed over the past three decades. Figures from Scotland (*The Scotsman*, December 2015), for example, reported that teachers across Scotland had taken more than one million sick days over the past three years. The data on teacher illness in primary and secondary schools revealed that the 343,330 sick days in 2015 was at a three-year high after increasing on the previous 12 months, with stress noted as a common reason for absence. A further breakdown of the figures showed that more than 20% of absences in Glasgow in 2015 were for 'psychological' reasons while in Edinburgh, stress and similar conditions accounted for 18.5% of absences.

Occupational stress

The prevailing feeling within the teaching profession in the UK has, for a number of years, been one of low morale and poor self-image. Educators are known to be overwhelmed with work and see 'Initiative Overload' from successive governments and agencies as being at the root of the problem, allied to the huge increases in bureaucracy and the mountain of paper work that this generates. In addition, educators have found that they are expected to take on greater and greater responsibility often very early in their careers (Martin, 2003). Posts of special responsibility, after-school activities, league sports teams, music or drama events, and the integration of children with special educational needs and disability within mainstream schooling, all create additional pressures for the teacher. As a result teachers are, in increasing numbers, bowing out. Figures published by the National Association of Head Teachers reported in 1994 that since the early 1980s, the number of teachers ending their careers early because of ill health trebled in the UK, with only one teacher in five working on to the statutory retirement age. Ofsted's annual report for 2002 found that there were real problems not only in recruiting but also in retaining teachers, with 20% of teachers leaving within their first three years in the profession; heavy workload was cited as one of the reasons for leaving.

Almost a decade and a half later the situation is no better, with a report in October 2016 noting that a third of teachers left the classroom within five years of qualifying, an increase of 13%; about 30% of the 21,400 who joined state schools in November 2010 had left the profession by 2015. The Head of the National Union of Teachers said that 'schools have become more difficult and less rewarding places to work'.

There is increasing evidence of a crisis in teacher recruitment and retention just as the number of pupils and the demand for new teachers begins to increase sharply. Excessive workload and attacks on pay are driving teachers away and deterring new recruits. A report in *The Sunday Times* (Henry and Griffiths, 2017) noted that schools are offering duvet days, golden hellos of £1,000, gym membership, and shopping vouchers in a bid to attract staff, as teacher training targets in England have been missed in most subjects for five years.

The physiological effects of stress

Stress may be seen to be an adaptive response by the body to changes in the environment, e.g., if confronted by a man-eating lion, most individuals would be activated by an instinctive response either to turn and run away or to stand and fight. Although evolutionary changes have made it less likely that individuals will meet many lions, the response to potentially threatening situations remains the same and the primitive body in a state of high alert prepares to use reserves of energy to 'fight or take flight'.

The threat of physical, emotional and psychological pain is ever present, if not actually encountered, and on occasions the 'fight-or-flight' response is triggered without the individual being fully aware of it; nevertheless, physiological change will have taken place. It is this physiological change that has, both directly and indirectly, an effect on the vocal process.

Stress is not, as has been noted, always negative; it can provide some health benefits when experienced in small amounts. The advantages of stress include an increase in motivation, a warning sign that there is something wrong and an increase in heart rate. Stress is able to provide a small burst of energy to people who are feeling unmotivated. It can be the push that some people need to get the day or a specific project started. People who are under small amounts of stress will be pushed harder to accomplish a project or finish something that needs to be done. Stress is, however, a warning that something is amiss, that those who are feeling too much stress may need to make a change.

Stress can increase the heart rate and can cause a slight rise in the blood pressure. For a heart to remain healthy, these increases are sometimes necessary. Stress can also increase the immune system by allowing it to function on a 'fight-or-flight' response for as long as is necessary. When, however, teachers and lecturers complete their term's or semester's work they often report that they then succumb to colds and illness as soon as the pressure of the job recedes and the fight-or-flight response is 'switched off'.

Some of the physiological changes that occur as the body, responding to the threat, 'prepares for action', regardless of how dramatic or otherwise this action is, are listed here:

- The pupils dilate and the mouth goes dry.
- The neck and shoulder muscles tense.

- The large skeletal muscles contract for action.
- Breathing becomes faster and shallower.
- The heart pumps blood faster so that blood vessels dilate.
- The liver releases stored sugar to provide fuel for quick energy.
- Digestion slows down or ceases.
- Muscles at the opening of the bladder and anus are relaxed.
- Cortisol, adrenaline, and noradrenaline are released.

Too much stress can weaken the immune system, so it is important that when the source of the threat is removed or resolved, the body returns to a stable state, or homeostasis. However, in a period of prolonged stress individuals may activate the stress response but cannot activate the accompanying physical response, becoming instead impatient, angry and irritated. These individuals do not, therefore, return to a stable, relatively constant state and it is in the inhibition of the physical response to stress that the danger to health lies.

Many of the stress-induced physical changes that have been described above will have a significant effect on voice quality. Reviewing these physical changes reveals a clear link between voice and stress:

- Difficulty in swallowing leads to a fixed laryngeal position, resulting in the voice losing flexibility and nuance.
- An aching neck leads to tension within the internal and external muscles of the larynx, resulting in loss of free movement of the vocal folds and limiting vocal range.
- Backache affects the easy movement of the ribs, resulting in a reduction in lung volume and breath support for voice.
- Muscle tension similarly affects the easy movement of the ribs, so lung volume is reduced and vocal support is compromised.
- Muscle tension reduces the flexibility and muscularity of the respiratory process.
- Muscle pain leads to reduced voluntary movement, resulting in stiffness and loss of flexibility, both of the ribs and the vocal folds.

- Fatigue leads to loss of effective muscle function and a consequent reduction in the flexibility and easy movement of the vocal folds, reducing pitch range.
- Frequent urination and diarrhoea lead to dehydration and a consequent effect on the vocal folds, producing a hoarse or rasping sound.
- A less efficient immune system leads to lowered resistance to upper respiratory tract infections and the potential for infection within the larynx, leading to changes in the mass of the vocal folds, which affect vocal pitch and range.
- Overly rapid shallow breathing leads to a reduction in both breath support and phonation time, resulting in a poor quality of voice.
- Indigestion may lead to gastro-oesophageal reflux, which will directly affect the vocal folds, causing redness and irritation and a change in the quality of the sound.

Examination of these physical changes in the light of the processes that affect voice illustrates the fact that stress may affect every aspect of phonation, including breath capacity, muscle function, reduced lubrication of the vocal folds, changes within the lining of the vocal tract and tissue integrity of the vocal folds. Although noting the physiological changes caused by stress, it is also important to recognize that the physical changes that occur in a state of low esteem will also contribute to vocal change. Here, the most noticeable changes are often postural, with lowered eye levels, slumped shoulders, rounded back and a much more contained, introverted posture, with accumulated tension in the shoulders, neck, and jaw.

As well as impacting on the quality of voice these cumulative changes, both physiological and psychological, occurring as a result of stress will often have the effect of making the individual feel exhausted and unable to function effectively. Later chapters explore language use within the teaching environment but it is important to note that although the focus here has been on the effect of stress on vocal quality, the use and retrieval of language may also be affected. Continually being studied and defined and not yet completely understood, language is a highly complicated process, paradoxically most vividly illustrated when there is a breakdown in the structure, for example, when an individual has a 'stroke'. The expression 'I was so tired that I could hardly say a word', more usually thought of as referring to the physical process of articulation, also encompasses the cognitive processes involved in 'saying a word'. Forgetting perfectly simple words or losing the train of thought is often aggravated by tiredness and, in some instances, tension and stress, which in turn produces adrenal fatigue.

Coping with change

Education is a dynamic political arena, the focus of government initiatives and funding, but for those at all levels within education, this dynamism can also be the focus of tension and stress. Teachers experience a sense of dislocation because the framework within which they teach changes. Syllabus changes will mean that teachers have suddenly to learn new material and often feel uncomfortable with the short period of time that they are given to assimilate it. Teachers who are qualified to teach one subject find themselves having to teach another with which they are comparatively unfamiliar, having to 'keep one step ahead' of the class. This is not to suggest that teachers want to collude in offering less than expert tuition but simply, that limits imposed by the staff:student ratio and the subject choices made by students mean that this does occur. The level of tension that is engendered is considerable; most teachers want to be prepared, to be confident about their subject and to feel that they can legitimately be the 'expert'. The difficulty for teachers lies in trying to reconcile the demands of the school administration and their own needs, and on most occasions the requirements of the school take precedence.

Within a small-scale study of newly qualified teachers and lecturers (Martin, 2003), respondents reported that they had been asked to take on additional roles of special responsibility for which they felt unprepared. If one assumes that these are not isolated cases, there must be many teachers struggling to maintain their position against overwhelming administrative and professional demands. In addition to voice problems relating to these demands, teachers frequently report voice problems related to classroom discipline or indeed, to incidents with individual pupils. Added to these professional demands, teachers are not immune to the effects of stress within their personal lives, e.g., bereavement, pregnancy, divorce, redundancy of a partner or a prolonged chronic illness, issues which do not prevent them from teaching but do have a very debilitating effect.

Stress and exhaustion

As has already been noted, for some individuals stress is stimulating and exciting, whereas for others a similar degree of stress is insupportable and can result in sleeplessness, depression, anxiety attacks or a vocal problem. Whether stress is stimulating or insupportable, both responses activate (as part of the fight-or-flight response) the release of large amounts of adrenaline and noradrenaline, which help individuals to maintain a high level of activity, giving that extra 'buzz' that people experience when working at full stretch. The effect, however, of unusually high levels of noradrenaline ultimately leads to an abrupt loss of energy, often accompanied by an overwhelming feeling of exhaustion unrelated to physical effort. Some educators experience this effect at the end of every term; for others, this is an occasional episode triggered when the cumulative effects of personal and professional stress become too much.

Changes in vocal quality

The effect of stress on the voice has already been outlined; the tired and strained vocal quality with which educators present at the end of term is a well known phenomenon in staff rooms all over the world. So too is the fact that many experience problems at the beginning of the autumn term when returning after a long summer break. One reason for this may be that during the long holiday period, educators have been able to affect some form of 'damage limitation' as far as the voice is concerned, by relaxing over the break and being released from administrative duties, student contact and teaching pressures. Periods of speaking with less effort and in a more vocally friendly environment allow the voice to return to a more natural vocal setting. The teacher returns to the school environment still using this 'holiday' vocal setting, but may soon find that the voice is inadequate for the teaching task and there is a need to readjust and adapt to the school/college environment.

Our individual response to stress and tension cannot be absolutely anticipated; we can predict areas of 'danger', but we do not know definitely what the effects will be. Some educators can demonstrate amazing vocal resilience for years, only to find that their voice disappears without any apparent increase in vocal loading. Others experience mild vocal symptoms for years that never get any worse or become unmanageable. What is known, however, is that most educators will describe similar symptoms: diminution of vocal flexibility, range, loudness or ease of voicing leading to an erosion of their concept of self. The inability to express feelings, emotions and thoughts properly because of voice loss caused by vocal misuse is very alienating.

Environmental factors

How can educators better anticipate factors that will increase the likelihood of vocal strain? Potential stress triggers and identified emotional and physical factors that can affect voice quality have already been discussed, and **Chapter 6** explores ways in which the voice can be protected.

Overcrowding

The influence of environmental factors as a source of stress may, however, be overlooked. It is important that teachers acknowledge the influence of the environment in which they work on their mental health – issues such as overcrowding and lack of personal space within the school. Well documented evidence shows that where individuals have to live and work in overcrowded conditions, levels of tension rise and this increase is reflected in heightened feelings of aggression and violence. A survey in the UK for the Association of Teachers and Lecturers (ATL) union reported that four out of 10 teachers had experienced violence from pupils in the year 2015, (BBC News education and social affairs, 29 January, 2016). Of those who had experienced violence, 77% said they had been pushed and around half were kicked or had an object thrown at them; nine out of 10 staff had dealt with challenging behaviour, such as swearing or shouting, in the past year. The government said that staff have greater powers to deal with poor behaviour, but 45% of the 1250-strong panel of teachers surveyed across England, Wales and Northern Ireland said they felt pupil behaviour had got worse in the past two years.

For many teachers, issues of overcrowding are considered only in terms of class size. Increases in class size are cited as giving teachers problems related to actual teaching efficiency. How can you teach 40 children in one class? How can you respond to the needs of every child? How can you keep control? There is also the issue of overcrowding and psychological response. It is clear that if one adds feelings of tension arising from overcrowding to the difficulty of controlling large numbers of children, the resulting cocktail is fairly potent.

Educators deserve to have some professional advice in terms of the new developments in ergonomics, and to try to limit problems of overcrowding if at all possible. Apart from the central issue of too many people in too small a space, it is also important to look at the effect that it has on students and learners who are equally influenced by the space in which they work. Educators report on the negative effect that the absence of a designated personal space has. This is particularly a problem for those in further education who are contracted, not to a college but to an agency, or for those individuals who work as supply teachers. Neither group has the luxury of a defined area in which they can work; in fact they have to carry their work space with them wherever they go.

Research indicates that individuals want to have a sense of a 'home' or a workplace with a designated space which they identify as their own territory. Many individuals like to mark their space with personal items such as family photos, books, etc. Without this personal space, teachers and lecturers can easily feel more separate and distant from colleagues, thus contributing even more to feelings of stress and tension. The environment in which an individual works or learns has a powerful influence on mood and emotion, one that should be considered more robustly. This highlights the importance of investing in a staffroom that provides comfort, warmth, and relaxation.

Work/life balance

The importance of achieving a satisfactory work/life balance has received and continues to receive considerable attention. A satisfactory work/life balance is the concept that suggests that individuals should endeavour to divide their time and energy between work and the other important aspects of their lives. Achieving work/life balance requires a daily effort to make time for family, friends, community participation, spirituality, personal growth, self-care, and other personal activities, in addition to the demands of the workplace.

Work/life balance is obviously greatly aided by an employer's willingness to institute policies, procedures, actions, and expectations that enable individuals to easily pursue more balanced lives.

The pursuit of work/life balance reduces the stress that employees experience. When individuals recognize that they are spending the majority of their days on work-related activities while feeling as if they are neglecting the other important components of their lives, stress and unhappiness result.

Working hours

It is, however, difficult to fully reconcile differing demands such as a personal, professional and monetary need to work,. This is particularly difficult for educators who, it is acknowledged, work more intensively than people in many other occupations, with 50- to 60-hour weeks the norm. A survey in 2013 suggested that secondary head teachers worked on average 63.3 hours per week – the longest of any of the teaching jobs. Primary classroom teachers worked longer hours – 59.3 hours – than their secondary school counterparts who worked for 55.7 hours per week. The hours in a secondary academy were slightly less, at 55.2 hours. The survey suggested, however, that teaching hours are a minority of the workload, as a primary school teacher will spend on average 19 hours a week of timetabled teaching. It is a similar situation for secondary school classroom teachers, averaging 19.6 hours. Teachers' unions have warned about excessive workloads and complained about staff being put under too much pressure. For educators, the long working week (one of several grievances that have prompted teachers to go on strike) makes achieving a work/life balance challenging and so for many, stress is an inevitable part of their professional role.

Strategies to mitigate stress

Strategies to mitigate or 'cope' with stress, known as Stress Moderator Variables, are resources, skills, behaviours and traits that can reduce the negative impacts of stress. These may take the form of a range of interventions, from physical exercise to social support, that can help protect someone from the negative effects of a stressful life event such as loss of a job. Positive strategies for coping include proactive, meaning-focused and social activities such as exercise, new hobbies or meditation, which can all be good ways of relaxing. Cognitive Behavioural Therapy is offered by the National Health Service in the UK as an effective solution to stress and anxiety. These variables have been shown to lead to better outcomes in times of stress compared with someone who experiences the same life event without adequate coping skills or support. Obviously every person is different and may find that certain strategies work better than others, but when feeling overwhelmed, it's always helpful to reach out to others for support.

Locus of control

Insight into habitual stressors in relation to one's personal and professional life may be useful. According to Rotter (1966), locus of control can affect a person in their decision to adopt a health behaviour. He suggests that individuals with a strong internal locus of control (a belief that events in their life derive primarily from their own actions) tend to praise or blame themselves and their abilities in respect to life events. This self reflection and blame can add greatly to their levels of stress when things 'go wrong'. Individuals with a strong external locus of control (a belief that their decisions and life are controlled by environmental factors which they cannot influence, or that chance or fate controls their lives) tend to praise or blame external factors in respect of life events. Trying to regain control for these individuals is an important element in reducing stress when things 'go wrong'.

Self efficacy

Self efficacy, or the individual's belief about their capabilities, determines how they think, motivate themselves and behave. Self efficacy and self esteem are linked to locus of control and have been proved to have the ability to predict several work outcomes, specifically, job satisfaction and job performance. (Judge *et al.*, 2002, argue that the concepts of locus of control, neuroticism, self-efficacy and self-esteem measure the same single factor.) Under stress, as noted earlier in the chapter, self efficacy may become skewed and it is important to meet with others either in work or outside to objectively reaffirm one's capabilities.

Self control

Self control is affected by the emotional brain and under stress, the part of our brain that controls temper (the amygdala) can be bypassed, leading to emotional 'meltdown'. Be aware of how you are feeling and develop ways of releasing emotional tension through physical activity.

Anxiety

Excess anxiety can manifest in a number of ways. As noted earlier it can affect mental processing, so try to be aware that anxiety may cause you to jump to conclusions before understanding exactly what has occurred, be this related to a professional or a personal issue. Make sure that you inform others of stressful situations or when you are in a state of anxiety. Do not try to protect others by 'soldiering on'.

Experience

Rely on life experience, both personal and professional, to deal with stressful situations. For example, recognize personal issues triggered by stress and ask yourself:

- Are you drinking more?
- Are you doing less exercise?
- Are you eating more?
- Are you more short-tempered?

- Are you sleeping normally?

As an overarching strategy for dealing with stress the following solutions may be useful:

In relation to other people
- If possible encourage colleagues to form small self-help groups to problem manage and share ideas.
- Bring stressful situations to the notice of the people involved.
- Discuss various ways of dealing with stress with your colleagues.
- Give them the opportunity to deal with stressful situations openly and honestly.

In relation to yourself
- Practice stress management techniques such as:
  - a quick walk outside;
  - a physical workout;
  - meditation; and
  - mindfulness training.
- Create and sustain strong social support networks such as friends and interest groups outside of the work environment.

In relation to your environment
- Use the power of visual stimuli to alter the physical environment in which you work:
  - put up calming and motivating classroom posters;
  - if you are allowed, alter the colour of your teaching rooms, use calming colours of green and blue;
  - introduce soothing background sound by way of taped music; and
  - try to avoid spending long periods of time under harsh light.

Time management
Time management and task prioritization are key strategies in response to a growing recognition of the increased and unacceptable level of work overload

within many different working arenas in the UK, yet they are very difficult to achieve without help. Suggestions for better time management are:

- Working with another person to look at issues of concern.
- List making.
- Using a memo or day book in which to write all tasks and carrying forward those that have not been completed to the next day.
- Focusing on different approaches to administrative tasks.
- Remembering that it is impossible to get everything done.
- The most effective method is to learn to say 'no', taking care that this decision does not simply shift the load from you to another colleague with equal workload and responsibilities.

Workshops on stress and time management are to be recommended as a productive way of spending in-service funds, empowering the teacher and lecturer to make constructive changes to their personal and working environment.

Chapter outline

- Prevalence of stress
- Definition of stress
- Factors in stress
- Prevalence of teacher stress
- Occupational stress
- The physiological effects of stress
- The effect of stress on the voice
- Coping with change
- Stress and exhaustion
- Changes in vocal quality
- Environmental factors
- Work/Life balance
- Working hours
- Strategies to mitigate stress
- Time-management

References and further reading

American Institute of Stress. Available at: <https://www.stress.org/workplace-stress/> [Accessed August 2017].

Day C and Smethem L. 2009. The effects of reform: Have teachers really lost their sense of professionalism? *Journal of Educational Change* **10**(2): 141–57.

Department for Education. 2016. *Education and Training Statistics for the United Kingdom.* Issued 10 November 2016. Available at: <https://www.gov.uk/government/uploads/system/uploads/attachment_data/file/567019/SR54_2016_AdditionalText.pdf> [Accessed August 2017].

Department for Education – Statistics. 2017. *Initial Teacher Training.* Available at: <https://www.gov.uk/government/statistics/initial-teacher-training-trainee-number-census-2016-to-2017> [Accessed August 2017].

Department for Education – Statistics. 2015. *National Statistics – School Workforce in England: November 2015*. Available at: <https://www.gov.uk/government/statistics/school-workforce-in-england-november-2015> [Accessed August 2017].

European Agency for Safety and Health at Work. 2009. *European Risk Observatory Report EN 9. Stess at work – facts and figures*. Available at: <https://osha.europa.eu/en/tools-and-publications/publications/reports/TE-81-08-478-EN-C_OSH_in_figures_stress_at_work> [Accessed August 2017].

Health and Safety Executive. 2016. *Labour Force Survey 2016*. Available at: <http://www.hse.gov.uk/statistics/causdis/stress/stress.pdf> [Accessed August 2017].

Henry J and Griffiths S. 2017. Desperate schools woo teachers with duvet days and £1,000 *The Sunday Times*, 2 April 2017.

Judge, TA., Erez A, Bono JE, and Thoresen CJ. 2002. Are measures of self-esteem, neuroticism, locus of control, and generalized self-efficacy indicators of a common core construct? *Journal of Personality and Social Psychology* 83(3): 693–710.

Lightfoot L. 2016. Nearly half of England's teachers plan to leave in the next five years. *The Guardian*, 22 March 2016. Available at: <https://www.theguardian.com/education/2016/mar/22/teachers-plan-leave-five-years-survey-workload-england> [Accessed August 2017].

Martin S. 2003. An exploration of factors which have an impact on the vocal performance and vocal effectiveness of newly qualified teachers/lecturers. PhD thesis, University of Greenwich.

Milne S. 1999. Job insecurity leads to stress epidemic. *The Guardian*, 5 January 1999. Available at: <https://www.theguardian.com/uk/1999/jan/05/4> [Accessed August 2017].

Rotter, J. 1966. Generalized expectancies for internal versus external control of reinforcement. *Psychological Monographs* 80(1): 1–28.

Smit B. 2003. The emotional state of teachers during educational policy change. Paper presented at the *European Conference on Educational Research*, at the University of Hamburg, Germany, 17–20 September 2003.

The Scotsman. 2016. Available at: <http://www.edinburghnews.scotsman.com/our-region/edinburgh/teacher-stress-soars-by-10-across-city-s-schools-1-4257082> [Accessed August 2017].

Travers CJ and Cooper CL. 1993. *Teachers Under Pressure*. London: Routledge.

Weale S. 2016. Almost a third of teachers quit state sector within five years of qualifying. *The Guardian*, 24 October 2016. Available at: <https://www.theguardian.com/education/2016/oct/24/almost-third-of-teachers-quit-within-five-years-of-qualifying-figures> [Accessed August 2017].

Wu J. 1998. School work environment and its impact on the professional competence of newly qualified teachers. *Journal of In-Service Education* 24(2): 213–25.

5

Voice as a physical skill

When the voice is used to communicate it is not just the larynx and the organs of speech that are involved in the process but the whole body. Chapter 2 highlighted the many muscles used in the production of sound. In addition to these muscles the spine, and the relationship of the pelvis, ribcage, head, neck and shoulder girdle to the spine, have a significant effect on the voice.

This sense of the involvement of the whole body in the production of voice is not always appreciated, partly because the significance of the link has not always been well defined and partly because an accurate sense of physical self is not generally well developed. Asked, for example, to close their eyes and, using the hands, indicate the width of their hips, head or waist, or the length of the foot, individuals will generally overestimate the size. There is also often a mistaken assumption by individuals that they are taller or shorter than they actually are, even when judging height in comparison with others who they know well. Some individuals have little concept of themselves within space; they duck unnecessarily when passing through doorways and, when asked to explore the space behind themselves, agree that this is an area that they do not generally consider they inhabit. There is a tendency for the same spatial levels to be used repeatedly. In an effort to inhabit, explore or reconfigure personal space, the following exercise is very effective: imagine being in a personal glass sphere and use hands to touch and explore the outer limits of it; in this way, open up greater spatial awareness.

The mind–body–voice connection

The voice is often considered as separate from the body but natural gesture shows us how connected both thought and voice are to the body. When we are relaxed and engaged in our conversations we have no problems with what to do with our hands or how to modulate the voice. Our emotional states are also expressed physically and in the voice. When the mind is under stress the body is too and the stress carries over into the voice. We experience difficulty with breathing, pitch is affected and rises or becomes strident, words are hard to find or remember, and we can become 'tongue-tied'. An in-depth under-standing of the effects of stress is given in **Chapter 4**.

An essential element in addressing voice problems is to consider the body. As well as the physiological impact on vocal quality, slumped alignment can be perceived as low status or negative. Standing in a positive open manner will generally be perceived by others as being positive, relaxed and high status and in turn, can change the way we feel. We need to address the way we stand and move and to identify our tension and where it is manifested. While focus on the body is fundamental, addressing mental attitude must be the starting point. The influence of the mind on the physical state requires this.

Language reflects this connection of mind and body. Sayings such as 'be brave, take it on the chin', 'keep your chin up', 'don't carry the world on your shoulders' are familiar, as are 'take a deep breath' and 'grin and bear it' in difficult situations when courage is needed. In situations that promote frustra-tion, feeling a sense of 'being lost for words', 'dumbfounded', 'speechless', or 'being so angry I could not speak' is familiar, as is the phrase 'having a lump in my throat' when sadness is felt. Reticent speakers are often referred to as 'tongue tied', whereas loquacious indiscreet people may be described as having a 'loose tongue'. Developing a sense of awareness about the mind-body-voice connection, spatial awareness, how we use our bodies when working, and how stress and tension impact on the voice, can only be beneficial.

How an awareness of the mind/body connection can help voice work

- Awareness is the first necessary step in changing habitual physical and vocal patterns.
- Changing mindset impacts on the body and changing body patterns impacts on the mind; therefore you can alleviate feelings of negativity or low stature by making small changes in your body language.
- Raising your awareness of how you might be seen by others allows you to make positive and beneficial changes to the way you are perceived.
- Understanding the connection gives you an element of control. It helps you to predict and prepare for stressful situations.
- Developing your understanding of body language allows you to read signs of tension and stress in others.
- Awareness allows you to make physical changes that can help with feelings of despondency, motivation, low status, fear, and tiredness.
- It also allows you to recognize when you are beginning to tire and are beginning to push the voice.
- Awareness can alert you to the fact that you are starting to display signs that you are under pressure or are feeling de-motivated. If for example, you notice your voice rising in pitch, you can stop and 're-pattern' your delivery.

Vocal culture

It is said that Western society has become very cerebral, with individuals becoming less active. In addition to this, much communication is now online rather than face to face. Language has become a means of expressing ideas and conveying information in contrast to the physical and emotional language of what are sometimes described pejoratively as 'less sophisticated' societies, whose cultures are more vocally liberated and who have maintained a strong tradition of song, dance and story-telling in their communities. Loud voices accompanied by expansive physical gestures tend to be considered flamboyant or excessive in certain countries. Lack of voice/body connection, combined with little understanding of the link between body and voice, can limit an individual's ability to recognize the early warning signs of a voice in trouble.

For many people the voice is simply a way of communicating thoughts. It is associated with the upper body and is often depicted as a 'speech bubble' coming out of the mouth. We associate voice quality as something we hear rather than feel. It is useful to begin to think of the voice emanating from the whole body and as vibration, which may be felt as well as heard. These vibrations can easily be experienced by placing a hand on the chest and 'humming' a sustained /m/, /v/, or /z/. Check that the head and shoulders remain relaxed.

Body alignment

Many vocal problems are the indirect result of a lack of balance in body alignment. This balance can be altered by a serious event such as a back injury or fracture of the ribs, resulting in unconscious restriction of movement in that part of the body to avoid discomfort. Other muscles may work harder to compensate for an injury. Similarly, foot, back, neck, shoulder or chest pain can restrict movement and alter posture. Even something as simple as a change of footwear – a change in the heel height of a pair of shoes – can tip the natural balance of the pelvis and thereby affect spine, head and shoulder alignment with a consequent effect on the voice.

The spine

As was noted in **Chapter 2**, the spine reaches from the head to the coccyx. It is made up of the vertebrae, between each of which are intervertebral discs which are cartilages that separate one vertebra from another and provide a cushion. The spine has a certain amount of flexibility and also has natural curves. The flexibility of the spine and its curves allows a range of movement to be undertaken without injury – the curves in the spine absorbing, for example, the shock of jolting and landing when jumping. The spine, most importantly, shields the spinal cord and the nerve fibres that come through the openings between the vertebrae. Often, the term 'straighten the spine' is used when correcting alignment, but it is important to retain the spinal curves and, without over-exaggerating or straightening them, for the spine to feel long. Figure 5.1 shows the necessary curves in the neck, thoracic and lumbar regions of the spine.

When the spine loses its natural length as a result of factors associated with illness or ageing, it is important to note that the ribcage, which is attached to the spine and houses the lungs, becomes depressed. This usually results in the slumping forward of the shoulders so that the entire 'front' of the body closes downwards and inwards. Space for breathing to occur easily, as well as the elasticity of the ribs, is therefore lost. At the top of the spine is the head, positioned on what is called the atlanto-occipital joint, the joint between the top vertebra and the bottom of the skull.

Sometimes, in old age, the voice loses its resonance and range as the spine stiffens, flexibility is lost and the

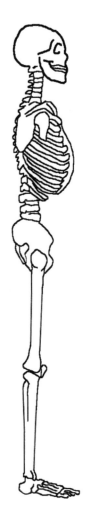

Figure 5.1: The spinal curve.

head pokes forward. William Shakespeare, in his speech about the seven ages of man, observes this:

> His youthful hose, well saved, a world too wide
> For his shrunk shank, and his big manly voice,
> Turning again toward childish treble, pipes
> And whistles in his sound.
>
> From: William Shakespeare, *As You Like It*, Act II, scene vii

105

What to do about posture and alignment

Ask yourself:

- How would others describe my posture? Would they say it was stooped, open, tense, over-corrected or collapsed? Standing in front of a fitting room mirror or looking at photographs can offer the answer. Ask a friend or partner to comment honestly.
- Are my shoes suitable and comfortable? Overly high heels can throw the body off centre.
- Is there any tension in my abdominal muscles?
- Does my back feel wide?
- Is my pelvis level or tilted forwards or backwards?
- Am I standing with weight balanced on both feet?
- Is my spine slumped or lifted?
- Is my spine long? Consider also the length of the back of the neck?
- Do I have an old or new injury that may be contributing to poor postural habits?
- How slumped or upright is my posture when sitting? Do I sit in a supported position at meetings or while relaxing?
- How much space is there between the base of my skull and my shoulders?

Helpful ways of re-patterning alignment

- Attend an Alexander Technique, Feldenkrais, Tai Chi, Qi Gong (also known as Chi Gong), Pilates, or yoga class, as all these improve awareness of alignment.
- See a doctor or appropriate health professional about physical injuries before surrounding muscles over compensate and problems develop.
- Check your posture while sitting at a computer or using a laptop, tablet and mobile/cell phone.

- Use reminders such as a brightly coloured spot on your fridge, land-line telephone, or in your car to remind you to make adjustments to habitual patterns.
- Mobile/cell phone alarm reminders or written notes on stickers can be equally useful.
- Adjust your posture after bending over desks.
- When carrying heavy books or other equipment, consider your spinal alignment.
- Avoid maintaining a hunched or awkward position for too long and always take the time to stretch the body regularly.
- Release shoulders after each session/class and at the end of the working day.
- If possible do release and alignment exercises with your students.

The head and neck

When asked how much they think the head weighs people offer a range of responses, from the very light 2 or 3 pounds, a little over a kilogram, to the much more accurate 12–15 pounds, or 6 kg. 'Guessing the weight of the head' has a serious intent, aiming both to impress on individuals the effort required to achieve a critical balance between the head, considering its heavy weight, and the neck and spine, and to consider what the implications of this are for the voice. If an item of similar weight was to be carried comfortably, it would quite naturally be held close to the body rather than at arm's length. Consider then the tension created when the neck is extended forward and the head, as a consequence, rather than being balanced easily on top of the spine is similarly extended so that critical head/neck alignment is lost. The effect of this is to recruit the large muscles of the neck, jaw and shoulders in order to compensate for this loss of alignment. This compensatory action is far reaching because, as has already been noted, there is a direct link between these muscles and the larynx. Proper alignment allows the body to move effectively and harmoniously without creating unnecessary tension.

Check your head/neck alignment frequently throughout the day, particularly at the start of a new class. Ask yourself the following questions:

- Are your ears positioned over your shoulders?
- Are your shoulders relaxed or raised?
- Is it possible to lower your shoulders?
- Is your neck free and flexible or tense and fixed?
- Could head thrusting be the result of undiagnosed short-sightedness?
- Are you maintaining a level gaze with peripheral vision?
- Is your head balanced and free to nod up and down with ease?

To illustrate this more effectively the following exercises are recommended:

1.	An excellent exercise for developing awareness in the top of the neck is that of the 'nodding dog' or 'marionette'. This exercise involves isolating the small muscles that allow the head to rock gently in a smooth, weightless manner, rather like the movement of the toy dogs once found on car dash-boards that have a head attached to the body by a large spring. As the car moves the head wobbles – a very similar movement is seen on the puppets in films of the Thunderbirds.

2.	Imagine a column of water is spouting up the spine and the head is floating on the top of it. Feel the weightlessness of the head.

3.	Making sure that the jaw is not clenched, try gentle 'yes' nods, then 'no' nods and finally try to use both in a 'nodding dog' movement. These take some practice but they give a very useful awareness to the occipital area at the base of the skull most involved in the 'fight-or-flight' response.

4.	Speaking a sentence, allow the head to nod gently on the spine like a marionette. Make all moves in slow motion first.

Figure of 8 Exercises

1.	To prepare for the exercise, which can be done sitting or standing, it is important first to relax the shoulders, neck, and jaw, and to feel length in the neck. Exercise the large muscles by drawing imaginary floor-to-ceiling lines using the nose as an imaginary pen. Start these lines at the right shoulder and move across to the left while drawing vertical lines a few inches or centimetres apart. This exercise allows the uppermost neck muscles, which contract in stress, to stretch and release.

2. Still using the nose as a pen, draw a figure of eight slowly and fluidly, first in the normal vertical manner and then as if it was lying on its side. Start at the centre point and move across and upwards to the right side while drawing a loop that then crosses the centre point and moves to create another loop on the left side. Continue this looping figure maintaining the flexibility in the neck. Stop if any dizziness or discomfort is felt.

The importance of eye levels

The physical effect that eye levels have on the body and therefore the voice is often under-estimated. Shy children and socially intimidated or depressed individuals often avoid eye contact and adopt a lowered head position. This has a domino effect: the sternum becomes depressed, resulting in a lack of openness in the ribs and pressure on the abdomen. As a consequence the individual is unable to achieve more than a very shallow breath, which in turn produces a monotonous vocal quality. The opposite of this is a rigidly fixed focus which tends to correspond to locked neck, clenched jaw and stiffly held shoulders, leading to a considerable amount of un-useful tension. This posture limits peripheral vision, because the eyes do not scan, but look fixedly ahead, giving an impression of aggression and rigidity. Tension limits the free exchange of breath and results in a vocal quality that is often strident, lacks flexibility and warmth, and can appear aggressive.

Open and balanced alignment encourages peripheral vision, and the individual is able to function within his/her world in an aware and integrated manner. These rather 'extreme' examples are included to signal the importance of posture not only in determining vocal quality but also in how an individual is perceived by others.

The shoulders

Most people will say they experience shoulder tension. The use of computers, lap-tops and tablets means that time is spent hunched over with heads jutting forward. Heavy bags are slung over one shoulder from early adolescence, and there is little time in busy lives to play sports that exercise and free the shoulders, as for example swimming. Emotional states impact on the shoulders to the point that our language has adopted sayings such as 'she has broad shoulders' to denote a facility or willingness to carry responsibility, or 'he is carrying the world on his shoulders' to suggest someone is depressed or anxious.

Although when released the shoulders are heavy, most of us habitually carry them just slightly higher than they are in a relaxed position. It is a good idea to release the shoulders frequently throughout the day as shoulder tension has a very real impact on the voice.

Shoulder release exercises

Do these exercises during breaks throughout the day. They can also be done with your students to release tension and calm them.

1. Place your right hand on your right shoulder and rotate the elbow as widely as you can first one way and then the other.
2. Repeat the same exercise on the left side using the left hand placed on the left shoulder.
3. With arms by your side, reach the hands down towards your feet. Feel the stretch in the shoulders. Hold the stretch for several seconds, then release and feel a greater sense of freedom in the shoulder girdle.
4. Shrug the shoulders up and then release them, taking care not to jar the neck.
5. Grasp your hands behind you and stretch the shoulders backwards.
6. Relax the shoulders and look ahead keeping the chin down. Suddenly stretch the arms backwards and downwards while opening the hands and spreading the fingers. Make sure the head and chin do not thrust forwards. Hold this stretched position while you breathe in

and out four or five times through the nose, then release. You should feel the front of the chest open.

Please note: classes will benefit from work on the neck and shoulders as learners and students often slump over desks while writing, reading or working on computers. They also carry heavy bags, often on one shoulder. Early intervention and attention to positive postural habits can reduce neck and shoulder tension in adulthood.

Unlocking the knees

An area of the body that is not immediately associated with voice is the knee area. Most individuals brace their knees in order to steady themselves, particularly when they are under stress. Those unused to the experience of public speaking or performing often remark 'My knees were shaking' or 'I went weak at the knees', which illustrates the body-mind connection and the ways in which tension and nervousness can manifest. When the knees are locked, a lower abdominal tension is created which interferes with diaphragmatic movement. For the breath to flow in and out of the body, it is important to stand in a balanced and open manner, with the knees released and gently flexed, the feet in contact with the floor, and the body arranged around the spine with the feeling that it is lengthened and wide.

The term 'lengthen' is often used in connection with posture. This comes from the Alexander Technique which teaches the need to gently oppose the force of gravity that seems intent on 'squashing' us downward and 'squeezing' us inward. The word 'oppose' is preferable to 'fight' because it does not bring with it images of over-correction. It is as common to find over-corrected, regimented posture as it is to find slumped, contracted posture; what is less common is the open, lengthened and wide 'ideal'.

It could be said that an individual's habitual posture is a measure of the way in which he responds to and handles the stress of daily living. Similarly, for many educators their posture reflects the stresses of the contemporary teaching environment. Some seem bowed by the volume of work and the seemingly

(a) 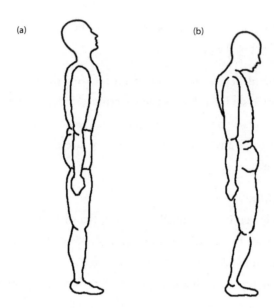 (b)

Figure 5.2: (a) Overcorrected position. (b) Slumped position.

insurmountable pressures; others take on the 'struggle' – literally – with chin thrust forwards and shoulders braced.

Exercises for releasing the knees

1. Standing, brace and then release the knees. Do this five times and then 'shake out' each leg.
2. With both knees together and slightly bent, reach down and hold the legs just above the knees. Rotate the legs in a circle, first to the right five times, and then to the left.
3. Raise the right knee up and then kick across to the left side of the body. Do the same with the left knee and then alternate the legs as if you were doing the can-can.
4. Tension held in the feet and ankles can transfer into the legs and knees, so it is always worth taking the time to stretch and release by pointing and circling the feet, much as is advised when flying.

Children's ability to shout without hurting the voice

Most primary school children in the playground are able to scream and shout during play time without losing their voices. There are a number of reasons for this: first, they tend to have natural alignment; secondly, they are playing so that their activities are free of harmful negative tensions (although no one would deny the positive tension involved in exuberant play); and thirdly, they are generally using the whole body and releasing the outgoing breath rather than holding it. There are of course exceptions to these generalizations: some children develop nodules or polyps on the vocal folds through improper use (Hunt and Slater, 2003) but they remain, fortunately, a minority of the school-age population.

Secondary school children present a very different picture. There is a considerable difference between the open and confident posture of the average 6-year-old and that of the average 16-year-old. When teachers are asked to demonstrate the posture of children in the class, boys are portrayed very differently from girls. When representing male posture, two very different stereotypical postures are portrayed: either the assumed confidence of the tight high-shouldered swagger, or a slumped spine body position with a concave chest, low eye level, with the head bowed in front of the shoulders. Girls are often portrayed as slumping forward with arms folded across the chest, or in some cases around the waist. In both boys and girls the significant similarity is the weight distribution. This is usually across one foot or hip, not two, resulting in a loss of space between the lower ribs and the hips, limiting the ribs' ability to widen, increase breath capacity and support the voice through expansion of the lower lung area.

Changes in adolescence

Just why this change from easy open posture and alignment to tight, contracted or slumped stance often occurs in the adolescent years, and in some cases the pre-adolescent years, is a complex subject open to much discussion. It is obviously the result of a number of factors. As children grow, particularly if they have a sudden 'growth spurt', they may temporarily lose some motor control and can appear ungainly, e.g., they may walk into objects or stub their toes. The way that they feel about themselves and their developing bodies can make them feel vulnerable and exposed. Much of the body language seen is an attempt either to protect themselves by withdrawing from society and making themselves inconspicuous by occupying as little space as possible, or assuming a postural confidence that they do not feel by lifting the shoulders, thrusting the jaw and taking up a greater amount of physical space. During this period, holding eye contact in everyday communication may be extremely difficult; this is because some young people cannot bring themselves to confront others, so their eye level tends to be lowered, thus producing the head/neck alignment that develops a slumped spine and results in shallow breathing.

In some teenagers it is possible to see the development of the use of head, neck and jaw in conveying the body language of either aggression or fear.

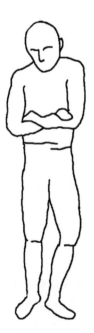

The threatening body language of the forward thrust jaw or the low eye levels found in the fearful and insecure is familiar. These ancillary movements of the neck, shoulder and head in response to fear and anger are a consequence of the 'fight or flight response' also referred to as the 'startle' effect by teachers of the Alexander Technique.

If possible, it is important to promote open and confident postural habits in the young by encouraging outdoor play and countryside pursuits, sport, drama and dance in order to counteract the negative postural effects of increased inactivity, social media, cell/mobile phones, and other technology.

Figure 5.3: Slumped adolescent posture.

Adult habits

Adults seldom correct or change the habits of adolescence; postural and movement patterns have been set and these continue to provide a pattern for adult life. Even when trying to absorb new patterns of alignment, the body 'prefers' the old pattern because it identifies and is comfortable with it, often rejecting the new posture as 'wrong'. For this reason, should posture be suspected to be a contributing factor in a voice problem, it is a very good idea to seek advice and to work with the help of an 'outside eye'. Once again there are many people who can help, from physiotherapists, osteopaths, chiropractors, sports therapists, Alexander Technique and Feldenkrais teachers, to Qi Gong, Tai Chi, and yoga teachers.

It is important to find someone who is qualified to work with the body therapeutically; practical help and advice need to be directed towards recognizing the uniqueness of each individual and fulfilling individual needs. For this reason, the advice on alignment offers general principles, but working with a teacher in a 'hands-on' manner is strongly advised if possible. If, however, there is no alternative to working alone, some of the following suggestions may be useful.

Some useful physical strategies
Film/video

Posture, as has been noted above, is difficult to change because in spite of the fact that it may need correction, it is habitual and therefore feels natural and comfortable. It is very difficult for individuals to 'step outside themselves', to see themselves as others see them. A mirror although useful does not offer the profile or back view unless it is a fitting room mirror, but an excellent alternative is to use a video to record movement and habitual posture. Video provides accurate feedback for those who need to work on posture but do not really understand what adjustments need to be made.

Most mobile/cell phones are equipped with video, so it is an easily available option; however, it requires very sensitive handling due to issues of data protection. Only use video with the express permission of the individual concerned, and only use their own mobile so that they can determine with whom they want to share the video contents. It is important to view the video with objectivity (an essential first step in gaining awareness), noting aspects such as head/shoulder relationship and the natural but unexaggerated curves in the lower back and thoracic spine. Notice also whether the head is carried forward or easily balanced on the top of the spine. It is important that the information gleaned from videos is used to develop a sense of physical awareness in individuals, which in turn allows them to recognize how their body feels when aligned.

Spot reminders

A very successful way of re-patterning the physical memory is to use the simple method of applying small coloured spots to strategic points around the home, office or classroom. For example, as a reminder to relax the shoulders, a spot placed on your mobile/cell phone or on the wall near a landline telephone in easy view will act as a trigger, when speaking on the phone, to encourage you to check head, neck and shoulder positions.

Holding the phone between shoulder and head, while the hands are involved in other activities such as looking up references, cooking or writing, can also affect vocal quality. Other useful positions for spots are on a watch strap, the fridge door, or the edge of a computer screen or tablet, on the steering wheel of the car, on the edge of the classroom board or on the school piano.

Health and safety training

Many industrial and commercial businesses are investing in postural training because of the number of working days lost through back injury and issues related to health and safety regulations.

These health and safety issues also affect those working in education and cause ongoing health issues as well as lost working days. Similar training in schools, universities or colleges provided by a recognized physical therapist is strongly recommended and would help to prevent posture-related vocal issues from developing.

Some companies offer meditation, and physical relaxation classes, as well as stress counseling, in order to prevent lost working days. This topic is further developed in Chapters 3 and 4.

Effort levels

As highly motivated and dedicated individuals, many educators wish to convey their love of a subject and their enthusiasm to their learners. Restricted time, pressures to attain results and issues with discipline can mean that many drive themselves and operate on consistently high effort levels.

When stress levels are high, it is more difficult than usual to assess effort levels, a task that is not easy even when most relaxed. Effort levels are usually assessed as either high or low depending on intrinsic and extrinsic mood and demand levels. It is, however, useful to be able to gauge physical and vocal effort levels so that energy may be expended appropriately and not wasted unnecessarily – over-use and excess effort is tiring and unproductive. The efficient use of energy and effort depends on developing awareness of the degree of effort necessary for specific tasks and matching the effort to the demand. High volume and energy is not always the best way to impart knowledge or control groups. Individuals tend to operate on a habitual effort level which makes it difficult to recognize that the job could be done equally well, with less effort.

Suggested exercises

1. An easy exercise to help to familiarize individuals with their own effort levels is to shake hands in pairs. Person A asks person B to shake hands and then to rate his or her own handshake on an effort scale of 1–10. If, for example, they rate it at 7, A then asks B to shake at effort level 3 or 9, then return to 7, go down to 4, up to 8 and so on, until he or she has established a graduated scale of effort. The partners then change over and repeat the exercise. This exercise has a practical application for voice use as less effort can often be more effective.

2.   Start by sounding a well breath-supported /ah/ vowel with varying degrees of energy, moving up the scale from 1 to 10 and assessing the different vocal effort needed for each stage. In this way the individual will begin to have a more accurate understanding of the amount of vocal effort, either high or low, that is consistent with specific vocal demands.

3.   Once this is achieved, and the level of vocal energy is spontaneously allied to the effort level, the exercise can be extended to short familiar classroom phrases or instruction, e.g., 'put your books away now', or 'in our next lecture we will be considering the politics of the period', or 'next week we are looking at bricklaying'.

4.   The exercise can be adapted to explore how changes in volume can be achieved without reverting to pushing, shouting and creating physical tension. By exploring increasing and diminishing volume through breath support from low in the body, confidence in the control of effort can be achieved and applied to the classroom or playing field. Simply start speaking some prose, verse or a speech at a comfortable volume (decide where it sits on your scale) and increase or lower the volume after a while. Do not rush through this as it will create tension. You may be surprised at how different volumes require more or less breath support. Stop yourself if you feel your posture begin to tighten or 'fix'.

Movement for classes

Learners and students will benefit from being given opportunities to stretch and move frequently thought the day. The benefits of including movement in the curriculum are well documented. Even if this is not possible, movement and play should be integrated into as many classes as possible in order to aid learning, promote physical, mental and social wellbeing and release tension. Details of useful websites and publications focusing on movement in the classroom can be found at the end of the chapter.

Chapter outline

- The mind body connection
- Vocal culture
- Body alignment
- Children's ability to shout without hurting the voice
- Changes in adolescence
- Adult postural habits
- Useful physical strategies
- Health and safety training
- Effort levels

References and further reading

Feldenkrais M. 1991. *Awareness Through Movement*. New York, NY: Harper Collins.

Fiore N. 2014. The benefits of movement in schools. *The Creativity Post*. Available at: <http://www.creativitypost.com/education/the_benefits_of_movement_in_schools> [Accessed August 2017].

Gelb M. 1996. *Body Learning*. New York, NY: Henry Holt.

Literacy and Language Center Inc. Available at: <literacyandlanguagecenter.com> [Accessed August 2017].

Project Zero Classroom 2017. Harvard Graduate School of Education (Pedagogy of Play) Available at: <www.pz.Harvard.edu> [Accessed August 2017].

Summerford C.2009. *Action-Packed Classrooms, K-5, using movement to educate and invigorate learners*. Thousand Oaks, CA: Sage Publishing.

Vineyard M. 2007. *How You Stand, How You Move, How You Live*. New York, NY: Nation Books (Perseus Publishing).

6

Personal and classroom strategies for care and maintenance of the voice

There is much that can be done to reduce vocal misuse through the use of simple strategies. Chapter 3 discussed vocal 'early warning signs and symptoms' of which educators should be aware. This chapter explores some of the specific strategies that they, as professional voice users, can adopt to conserve and preserve their voice and prevent potential career-limiting vocal difficulties.

The current zeitgeist is the importance of the mind-body link, how the mind can affect the body in critical ways. As has been mentioned in Chapter 4, stress is a critical factor in the constellation of factors that can affect voice quality and vocal health, as is posture and postural issues. While their link with voice quality and vocal health have already been discussed in broad terms in Chapters 2 and 5, this chapter will look in much greater detail at classroom-specific postures that can become habitual and lead to chronic physical and vocal problems. An obvious problem arises from the extensive use of tablets, laptops and phones, not only for personal use but also in schools and universities. Research by Deloitte (2015) suggested that individuals check their mobile/cell phone on average 46 times per day. Although 46 checks per day was the average, that number varied depending on the user's age group. Those between the ages of 18 and 24 looked at their phones most often, with an average of 74 checks per day. Americans in the 25–34 age bracket looked at their devices 50 times per day, and those between 35 and 44 did so

35 times each day. This figure has since increased; a year later in 2016 a blog by Hallan (19th April 2016) suggested that an average smart phone user unlocks and checks his/her phone 80 times per day. Hallan suggests that assuming a person has a 12-hour usage, 'he or she might be unlocking and checking the iPhone 6–7 times per hour, like, every 10 minutes. If this seems excessive, there are users who unlock and check their iPhones at an even higher rate'.

Such significant periods of time spent looking down at smart phones or tablets inevitably compromises head–neck alignment. Apart from the generalized stiffness and discomfort experienced, there is also an impact on the voice as alterations in the head–neck–spine relationship and change to the position of the larynx within the pharynx can occur. This in turn can constrict the larynx and change the configuration of the pharynx and the vocal tract, leading to a rather 'squeezed' vocal sound.

The height differential between the height of the infant teacher and the height of the desks in infant school requires the teacher to spend sustained periods of time leaning over while speaking to children or marking their work (see Figures 1.1 and 1.2 in **Chapter 1**). If possible the teacher should crouch beside pupils or draw up a chair alongside the child when explaining or helping with work.

Some schools and colleges do not encourage staff to sit while taking lessons and indeed, many educators prefer to stand, but it is tiring and this tiredness can compromise vocal performance. It is therefore very important for educators to try to monitor their posture in different activities throughout the day, due to the close connection between the voice and the physical condition of the body. If the spine is out of alignment the ability to support the body without undue effort or stress is reduced. Good posture allows free muscular movement of the voice and respiration; the skeletal structure should support the muscular overlay, not vice versa.

Poor posture, be that sitting working at a desk or computer, standing and giving instructions to the class or during leisure time spent looking at email and social media accounts can affect the quality, volume, pitch and resonance of the voice. When the body is free from excess tension and the skeletal framework is able to find its natural alignment, breathing improves and the voice functions without restriction.

Good posture can be achieved equally well in a sitting position as in a standing position. The 'sitting' bones may be used in the same way as the feet to support and balance the body. An easy, upright but not rigid spine is important, as is opening up the thoracic area so that the ribcage is free and lifted. As noted above, today's increased use of technology as a feature of work and leisure encourages individuals to spend a considerable time sitting, leading to a 'slumped' position. This position constricts the mid-portion of the body that can lead to rib immobility and reduced breath capacity. The following postural considerations will help to avert potential problems.

Apart from the postural implications in terms of stress and tension sites, slumped and rounded posture has an effect on communicative intent; it portrays someone who appears to be lacking in authority. The professional 'persona' of the educator is highly dependent on their physical presentation; teaching is after all a 'performance profession' (Lemov, 2010). Physicality is therefore a very important marker in terms of establishing a 'first impression', as will be discussed more fully in **Chapter 7**. Posture reflects confidence, psychological state or wellness, plus issues of self-esteem and self–image. In addition, good posture provides support for the voice quite effortlessly, reducing the potential for vocal misuse.

Very small changes in posture can make a significant difference. For example, when working on relaxing the upper body, educators often report little awareness of an habitually high shoulder position. For many, a high shoulder position never alters, whether driving, reading, walking or sitting. By raising the shoulders, the space within the pharynx is limited and the larynx is constricted, so voice is produced much less easily. In Chapters 5 and 11 a range of exercises are suggested, several of which will help with postural change, but alongside exercise try to take time during the working day to consider and monitor your posture so that it becomes routine.

Systematic monitoring of your body posture can distinguish between what is normal and what has become habitual. Once identified, postural problems are not difficult to deal with and achieving a 'new' posture is often initially easy. The difficulty lies in maintaining change, which does take time and awareness. Considerable effort has to be expended to make the 'new' seem comfortable and until established, far from seeming better, posture may indeed seem rather worse. Consultation with an alignment professional such as an Alexander, Feldenkrais, yoga, or Pilates teacher may be the most effective way of changing poor habitual posture.

Sitting

As already noted, good posture can be achieved equally well in a sitting as in a standing position. The 'sitting' or ischium bones serve the same function as the feet and it is therefore important to remember to use these bones to provide adequate support and balance when sitting. Although classroom practice encourages educators to embrace movement rather than maintaining a fixed position it is important, if sitting for long periods of time, to pay attention to the seating provided. Seating in schools is not always comfortable and uncomfortable seating not only imposes back strain but also exerts pressure on the abdomen; when slumping forward breathing is restricted, when slumping backwards pressure is put on the lower spine. Chairs should offer adequate support for the back and should be at a good level when working at a desk.

As a guide:

- Chair height should allow an individual to reach the surface of the desk comfortably.
- When both hands are flat on the surface the arms should be bent at a right angle.
- When writing at a desk, table or keyboard, one of the first requirements is to use a sloped surface, which creates much less strain on the wrists (a piece of board, or a tray with a support behind it, can be used to make a sloped surface).
- When using a computer, the keyboard should be angled through the use of a support behind.

Reported incidents of, for example, repetitive strain injury (RSI) or postural and eyestrain problems through extended computer use have contributed to the development of rigorous health and safety documentation. This documentation, which is legally binding, should ensure that staff are protected in the workplace, so educational institutions will often purchase customized keyboards through their occupational health departments.

Educators have frequently been caricatured as individuals clad in academic gowns and weighed down by piles of books. Undoubtedly many educators do have to carry far too much material, particularly if they do not have an assigned work station or classroom and have to move around the school or college campus with teaching materials. Despite the use of email for home assignments and assessment, paper-based assessments are often marked at home and need to be carried out of school or college.

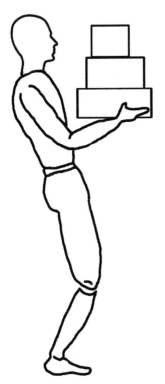

Within the classroom, large amounts of material need to be kept 'available' for projects, which involves the teacher moving boxes of stationery, equipment and project material from place to place. As with carrying heavy weights, the potential for damaging the lower back is high. The best way to carry heavy weights is close to the body, cradled against the chest or, if a substantial amount of material has to be carried, it should if possible be divided into two piles with the weight distributed equally, otherwise undue strain will be imposed on the spine and lower back

Educators with chronic pain or tension should if possible invest in themselves in terms of treatment. When the

Figure 6.1: Incorrect carrying position. problem is chronic rather than acute, a consultation with a qualified, licensed practitioner such as an osteopath, a physiotherapist or a chiropractor is recommended. Alternatively, working-with a qualified Alexander, Feldenkrais, yoga, or Pilates teacher, as has been suggested, can do much to improve the situation and prevent vocal problems resulting from poor posture. When muscles are damaged in some way (and problems in the neck, upper back or shoulder area can easily occur), an instinctive protective response is initiated and this, as noted in **Chapter 2**, can result in discrete changes within the skeletal and muscular framework that will affect voice.

Liquid intake

It is extremely important that the vocal folds are well hydrated in order to better withstand the intense demands of prolonged voice use. As a rough 'rule of thumb', the more an individual has to speak, the more he/she should drink, so teachers, lecturers and trainers should ensure that they keep hydration levels high to prevent dryness of the tissue and membrane of the vocal tract. It is also important to recognize that increased levels of hydration in the form of water should be introduced gradually, as the fluid takes some time to be absorbed and to hydrate the vocal folds. Prepare for a long speaking engagement or a period of heavy vocal use by increasing your fluid intake the night before, but the mantra of 'regular small amounts' should be remembered. Classrooms are frequently artificially dry and overheated yet teachers are often discouraged from drinking during class, not because of regulations imposed by the school, but quite prosaically because the result of drinking more means leaving the classroom and going to the bathroom. Recent concern about the levels of dehydration among learners and students, leading to reduced concentration and learning ability has, however, increased attention on levels of hydration, and it is hoped that improved focus on this will have a correspondingly beneficial effect for educators.

There remains some debate about the amount of fluid to drink on a daily basis but the authors' personal recommendation is at least 1 to 2 litres of water, bottled or tap, sparkling or still, per day, in addition to that contained in the normal intake of liquid through drinks such as tea and coffee. Tea and coffee have a diuretic effect and as such can be dehydrating, so it is important to 'top up' with water in order to maintain the moisture level within the body at an optimum level. Indeed some specialists would suggest avoiding tea and coffee completely and substituting herbal teas. The maxim 'pee pale' is a good rule to follow; urine that is pale in colour indicates a good level of hydration in the body. For those on medication it is important to remember that some medication (vitamin B, for example) can make urine darker in colour. Although drinking cannot directly lubricate the vocal folds, increasing fluid intake will 'top up' the general body fluid level and prevent dehydration. It is particularly important to keep the fluid level topped up when the vocal folds are in any way vulnerable. For example, in women of menopausal age, as was discussed in **Chapter 2**, the vocal folds are subject to tissue change, as are those in individuals who are heavy smokers or drinkers.

Many schools now have water dispensers in each classroom but if this is not the case it is most important for teachers to try to petition for one. Another solution is to introduce a cold water humidifier into the classroom to limit atmospheric dryness, subject to health and safety approval. Whatever the outcome, it is most important for educators to try to keep water to hand.

Educators who are working on the design and technology syllabus should make a concerted effort to remember to wear a mask if working on materials likely to create dust with lathes or saws. Small dust particles are very irritating to the vulnerable larynx, as are paints or varnishes. Teachers and coaches who are taking swimming classes in heavily chlorinated swimming pools should be vigilant in case of possible adverse reactions. Sensible health and safety guidance should ensure that teachers are provided with the requisite protection.

Steaming

In an effort to minimize some of the dryness experienced as a result of colds, vocal fatigue and stress, steaming is a very effective way of introducing moisture into the vocal tract. The tried and tested method of inhaling steam by leaning over a bowl of hot water (it is not necessary to add herbal extracts to the water) is very successful or alternatively, having a long shower remembering to inhale the steam, preferably through both the nose and the mouth.

A useful and perhaps more practical alternative is a nebuliser or steam machine, which allows moisture to bathe the vocal folds and reduces dryness in the respiratory tract. Nebulisers are currently available from high street pharmacists at a reasonably moderate price. It is important to remember that these machines must be cleaned out meticulously after use because fungal infections can occur if the machines are not properly and hygienically maintained. The use of distilled water is recommended and oils or herbal preparations should not be added to the machines. The authors' professional experience with occupational voice users suggests that maximum benefit is incurred by using the nebuliser three times a day for five minutes at a time. Steaming before giving a long presentation or performance is an excellent measure to prevent vocal damage/misuse. The effects of hydration on the vocal folds have been the subject of several well regarded studies (Verdolini-Marston et al., 1994), and many actors and singers use steam regularly to keep the vocal folds lubricated. Increased hydration levels will affect the speed and ease with which the folds move, which has an important effect on voice quality. It is also important to remember that in the process of vocalization, heat is generated by the action of the vocal folds; this increases dryness in the vocal tract and in combination with the drying properties of overheated classrooms, makes the workplace a very challenging vocal environment for educators.

Smoking

It is not the purpose of this book to proselytize on behalf of the anti-smoking lobby; the negative effects of smoking are well known, but perhaps less well known are the negative effects of smoking on the voice. Smoke irritates the respiratory tract and specifically affects the vulnerable vocal folds. Upper respiratory tract irritation, and sinus and asthma problems, can all be exacerbated by contact with smoky environments. In terms of vocal health it is important not to smoke, while the long-term impact of e-cigarettes, or 'vaping' has not been fully explored. It is encouraging to note that most schools and educational establishments are smoke free; others offer a separate smoking area. In the same way that smoking has an effect on the voice, so too do recreational drugs and cannabis.

Diet/reflux

Increasing importance has been paid to the effect of gastro-oesophageal reflux on the general condition of the vocal folds. This is where gastric acid from the stomach is regurgitated, spills into the larynx and bathes the laryngeal mucosa, resulting in irritation to, or inflammation of, the mucosal linings (Jones *et al.*, 1990). Any change to the structure of the vocal folds alters their vibratory characteristics, leading to change in vocal quality. In instances of gastro-oesophageal reflux, the structural change in vocal quality is perceived acoustically as hoarseness. This perception of hoarseness may encourage the individual to increase vocal effort in order to overcome the hoarseness and this in turn may compound the vocal damage.

Digestive problems may occur without an individual being aware of them, so undiagnosed and untreated gastro-oesophageal reflux may be present and not recognized unless specifically assessed as part of a full vocal assessment. In instances where gastric reflux has been identified, it is particularly important for individuals to avoid eating late at night in order to maximize the time spent during the digestive process in a vertical position. The distance between the upper end of the digestive tract and the larynx is approximately 20 cm so, in a prone position, there is more likelihood for gastric acid to seep into the larynx and cause inflammation and ulceration. One remedy is either to sleep on raised pillows or to raise the head of the bed. Spicy or highly seasoned food, fats, coffee, chocolate, smoking, alcohol and 'gassy' drinks can all aggravate the condition. It is important to be aware of food or liquid that is likely to cause adverse reactions and to avoid it if possible.

The effect of acid reflux on the vocal folds with associated voice quality changes may also occur as a result of frequent vomiting. Educators, parents, and carers should be aware that changes in voice quality might indicate a bulimic condition in young susceptible adolescents both male and female, as discussed in **Chapter 2**.

Various types of food may contribute to thickened saliva and dryness of the mouth. Spicy food, for example, may result in thirst and a dry mouth, whereas foods with high carbohydrate content, or thick milky sauces, often lead to sticky thick saliva. A dry mouth and thick secretions will encourage regular throat clearing, leading to irritation and potential damage to the vocal folds.

Throat clearing

Throat clearing and coughing are often the presenting symptoms of vocal abuse. Many individuals are quite unaware of how often they cough or clear their throats, but the sensation of having a 'frog in the throat' or a 'tickle' is one that is frequently cited by those with voice problems. Unfortunately, the process of 'clearing' the throat has quite the opposite effect because in coughing, the vocal folds are brought together with considerable force. In turn, the vocal folds, in an effort to reduce the ensuing friction, become bathed in mucus that the individual then feels the need to get rid of by clearing the throat, and so the problem continues. One way to limit this vicious circle is to keep a supply of water available and try to sip some water rather than clear the throat; the action of sipping the water appears to limit the need to clear the throat and gradually the problem becomes less acute. If it is not possible to sip water try instead to swallow, rather than cough.

Hard attack

Hard attack, where the vocal folds come together forcefully at the onset of a word beginning with a vowel, is the result of a lack of co-ordination between the initiation of voice and the initiation of breath. A common characteristic of the speech of stressed individuals, it manifests as a hard initial explosion of sound especially evident in phrases where words begin with vowels, such as 'All right Class 8, I said quiet!' The lack of synchronization of the muscles of breathing and the muscles of speech resulting in the vocal folds coming together with great force may, over a period of time, damage them. If this is an established habit it can be remedied by allowing a little breath through the vocal folds before speaking, e.g., adding a silent /h/ before the words 'all right' so that it becomes 'h-all right' takes the stress off the initial sound. (Make sure you say the sound of the letter /h/ not the name of the letter /h/.) Practice in saying lists of words beginning with vowels in this way encourages a more gentle onset of the note and helps the muscles of breath and voice 'remember' the appropriate posture and effort level required; once this action has become familiar, it should be enough simply to 'think' /h/ before vowels to reduce hard attack. Habitual vocal patterns tend to be strongly entrenched and therefore, in order to achieve vocal change, it is important to persevere with exercises for some time. Chapter 11 gives details of this and other onset exercises.

Projection

Projection of the voice allows the speaker to be heard in large spaces without amplification. Projection requires vocal range, clear articulation, and a desire to take command of the space and share the information with the audience. It is dependent on the ability to provide an adequate, unrestricted breath supply to fully support vocal fold movement without tension or constriction. A well aligned, open posture will allow specific resonators to give warmth, energy and volume to the voice. A common fault is to lock the neck, thrust the head forward and to shout, causing strain and a loss of clarity. Those listening then struggle to hear what is being said. When vocal projection is lacking the ability to assimilate information is impeded. It is also important to remember that personality and not just voice should be projected, and that this will create a greater connection with a class, group or audience.

Positive actions to be encouraged when addressing large groups in classrooms, lecture rooms and halls are:

- a sense of ownership of the space;
- a positive attitude to the audience and enjoyment in communicating;
- comfortable shoes and clothing;
- confident, balanced posture;

- an open and relaxed stance;
- weight well distributed over both feet;
- preparation of the breathing mechanism and vocal muscles;
- preparation of the material to be delivered (speech or lecture);
- adopt a confident physical status, with a friendly and relaxed attitude;
- released tongue, jaw, and shoulders;
- eye levels and eye contact that takes in the whole audience;
- relaxed and supported voice;
- range and musicality in the voice;
- familiarization of the space before meeting a class or giving a lecture; and
- well written and rehearsed material.

A raised platform may be helpful for audibility and might improve observation of the class and communication with the students. Further exercise on projection and working with volume can be found in **Chapter 10.**

Ventilation

A number of common causes of vocal misuse have their origins in environmental conditions endemic to academic life. Although it may not always be possible to change conditions, it may be possible to mitigate them by, for example, following certain rules of vocal hygiene and voice care. Educators frequently work in buildings where ventilation is a problem, often because the windows are hermetically sealed and cannot be opened, even partially. During winter, when the central heating is turned on, classrooms can become too hot, and a very dry atmosphere will affect the respiratory tract and the larynx. Air conditioning can have the same effect, so it is very important to be aware of the possible effects on the voice and to take steps to lessen the problems. Possible ways of doing so are to:

- make a case for improved ventilation on account of health and safety;
- ensure drinking water is always available;

- ventilate classrooms between sessions by opening doors and windows; and
- if the opportunity arises, take groups to suitable outdoor spaces.

Common classroom infections

Inadequate ventilation contributes to the spread of infection so that coughs and colds abound. It may be necessary to have a well-documented procedure for minimizing the spread of coughs and colds. A plentiful supply of tissues should be available in the classroom, which children should be encouraged to use.

Attempting to limit infection is important because repeated colds can be particularly debilitating, and many teachers report that their voice first showed signs of deterioration after a bad cold. The recommended vocal management in the case of a cold or respiratory infection is to:

- try to talk as little as possible at work and at home;
- take time off in order to recover if necessary;
- look after the voice by drinking plenty of water;
- steam the voice;
- rest the voice;
- minimize talking to the class throughout the day;
- indicate that you have a cold and need to talk less;
- establish a non-verbal control by using signs or sound; and
- set activities that can be achieved silently.

Cold remedies

Individuals anxious to avoid the need to take time off work frequently use over-the-counter cold remedies that are designed to eliminate excess moisture and 'dry up' a cold. These cold remedies contain a high level of caffeine, aspirin, and often antihistamines. They are certainly effective but, for professional voice users such as educators, the drying effect on the vocal tract, allied to the vocal demands of the role, is difficult to reconcile. There is always a conflict between taking time off work with what appears to be a rather trivial illness and 'soldiering on', but it is important to remember the damage that can result from 'forcing' the voice even for short periods.

If the voice is to be used strenuously and at a high volume over a period of time, it is advisable to use paracetamol and not aspirin as a remedy for colds and flu. The blood-thinning properties of aspirin can, in some circumstances, contribute to haemorrhaging of the vocal folds. Sucking throat lozenges and pastilles should be kept to a minimum, because they often contain strong dosages of decongestants that can affect the vocal tract. It may be worth noting that mentholated sweets that can be bought over the counter have a very limited effect on the mucosal lining of the nose, and although they may seem to 'clear' the nasal passages, they would appear to be more of a panacea than a cure. It cannot be stated too forcibly that any vocal change persisting for longer than two to three weeks after a cold should be reported to a doctor.

Allergies

Given the increase in over-the-counter medication it is not uncommon for individuals to self-diagnose and, without seeing a general practitioner, to self-treat for a variety of conditions including hay fever or common nasal allergies. For many, these remedies work well but for others, even a mild nasal decongestant may have a negative impact on the nasal mucosa. Frequent use of sprays for allergies, without advice from a pharmacist or general practitioner as to the pharmaceutical content, is not recommended. Professional voice users should ensure that medication is appropriate and does not have any unwanted side effects that may contribute to vocal attrition.

Clothing

Classrooms, school and college premises are extremely difficult to heat to a constant temperature. In the early morning the classroom is usually quite cool, with the temperature warming to a muggy heat by the time the last bell goes. As a result, teachers and lecturers often find that they are cold when they come into work and remain cold for some time after starting work, especially in older premises that are not well insulated. When cold, blood vessels contract to maintain as much body heat as possible and cold muscles do not work as efficiently as they do when warm. In an effort to conserve heat the tendency is to limit movement and indeed individuals may often be seen 'hugging' themselves to retain body heat. A useful tactic is to wear layers of clothing, so that as the room heats up a layer can be divested and a steady degree of warmth throughout the day can be maintained. Clothing that is too tight, particularly across the chest and back, can impede breathing by restricting the degree of rib expansion and in the same way, belts that are pulled too tight will constrict the diaphragm, particularly when individuals are seated, thereby limiting effective respiration.

Physical fitness

The link between voice and physicality has already been explored earlier and in **Chapter 5**, but it is important to remember that keeping flexible and mobile is very important, not only for long-term health but also in an effort to underpin and maintain effective respiration, reduce areas of tension and encourage vocal flexibility. Counteracting some of the effects of ageing on the skeletal framework is also to be recommended because effective and efficient use of the voice is possible into old age, providing that supple rib movement is maintained in order to aid respiration and conserve good spine, pelvis, head and neck alignment.

Yoga, Tai Chi, and Pilates classes are a particularly useful way in which to focus on relaxation, breathing, balance and general muscular flexibility. Low-impact aerobics, as well as encouraging physical fitness, will also contribute to increased respiratory function. Keeping fit has the additional benefit of releasing endorphins as well as discharging tension; endorphins influence mood and are generally thought to contribute to a feeling of well-being. For many people who find exercise classes tedious, a creative alternative form of exercise could be a dance class. If formal classes are not of interest, regular walking will improve breathing, strengthen muscles and bone, and improve stamina. Swimming will serve the same function and is particularly good for the muscles involved in respiration; swimming has the added benefit of being totally impact free, which is of relevance to the older individual and particularly relevant to those who may have osteoarthritic or rheumatic joint conditions.

Warming up

As with any form of intense physical activity it is important for educators to warm up vocally before beginning a day's teaching; the vocal equivalent to a marathon. Athletes warming up before a race are rarely seen running on the spot. Most perform an initial series of stretching exercises that gently encourage muscle movement and only then do they start to jog, or run slowly; never do they run at full stretch as part of their warm-up routine. Educators, however, once they begin work, rarely do anything but the equivalent of 'running at full speed' vocally. To spend time gently 'stretching' vocally and making contact with the breath is important.

Vocal warm-up leads to an increase in blood flow to the muscles and an increase in nutrient deposition to the muscles used. As a result, exercised muscles have increased activation potential and possibly improved fine motor control; in effect, they work better. The vocal warm-up exercises included in Chapter 12 are very useful preventive measures against vocal misuse, and are to be recommended. Warming up can be brief and subtle and can be carried out almost anywhere. Humming a tune gently and sliding up and down the range on the sound /n/ or /m/ is a low-impact vocal exercise that can be carried out almost anywhere, from sitting in the car to walking down a corridor.

A strategy for warming up is to involve the class (if the learners are of an appropriate age) by doing exercises that both relax and energize everyone. An all-over stretch is very beneficial and can be incorporated into classroom activities without disrupting the teaching routine. The stretch allows the children to alter their positions; this not only prevents them from getting stiff but at the same time releases tension, which might result in the children fidgeting and losing concentration. The stretch in fact re-focuses the children's attention and does not, as might be thought, prove distracting. Remember that postural habits can become fixed during pre-adolescence, so any input reaps the double benefit of helping the class and the teacher. There was a time when physical education in schools actively promoted postural awareness, and it is regrettable that this is no longer the case. Any individual effort on the part of the teacher should be seen as a bonus for students and learners.

Vocal care – individual responsibilities and strategies

The following checklist serves as a reminder of voice care recommendations.

Vocal care recommendations

- Do not try to talk above loud background noise at social or sports events, or above machinery noise.
- Avoid smoking.
- Avoid chemical irritants or dusty conditions.
- Avoid using recreational drugs.
- Try to keep alcoholic drinks to a minimum.
- Do not respond by shouting when upset or anxious.
- Avoid excessive use of the phone.
- Be aware that spicy foods and dairy products may affect your voice.
- The voice is closely linked with emotion and therefore vulnerable during times of tension or depression. Try to avoid extensive vocal loading at such times.
- The voice needs moisture – keep up your liquid intake.
- Pale-coloured urine indicates a good level of hydration.
- Steam when required and, particularly, when ill and before periods of prolonged speaking.
- Avoid dry atmospheres – use a humidifier or water spray to moisten the air in centrally heated classrooms, offices or homes; if you

---

have conventional sealed radiators a wet towel draped over the radiator effectively humidifies the air.

- If your voice is hoarse or you are losing your voice, do not whisper or try to continue talking; rest your voice.
- Remain vigilant in terms of your voice quality.
- Monitor any change in your voice carefully and see a doctor if there is a persistent change in quality.
- If you are experiencing continuing vocal problems, ask your GP to refer you to an ENT specialist or otolaryngologist.
- If you are prescribed new medication be aware of any changes to your voice quality, or any aspects that might cause irritation to your vocal folds, such as an increased tendency to cough or to feel dehydrated.
- If you suffer from hay fever and need antihistamines be aware that they can cause dryness to your vocal folds.
- Some cold and flu remedies may also 'dry out' the vocal folds so monitor your voice carefully if taking these over-the-counter medications.
- Warm up the voice gently before prolonged speaking.
- Try to sip water or swallow if you feel you need to clear your throat as vigorous throat clearing will damage your vocal folds.
- Try not to wear tightly fitting clothing that restricts your ability to breathe deeply. Wear layers of clothes so you can respond to the ambient temperature in the work place and avoid getting too cold or too hot.
- Try to keep physically fit and mobile in an effort to maintain effective respiration, reduce areas of tension and encourage vocal flexibility.
- Try to avoid bringing the vocal folds together forcefully as this 'hard attack' at the beginning of words can damage the vocal folds.

Hearing

Teachers will all be familiar with the problem of hearing impairment in pupils. This may range from a degree of hearing loss that requires hearing aids, to intermittent deafness caused by recurrent middle ear infection (otitis media), commonly known as 'glue ear'. For some primary school children this can be a source of continual absence from school and indeed, because of the fluctuating nature of middle ear infection, a child may be able to hear clearly one day and not the next. As noted previously, speech and language disorders ranging from relatively minor problems to much more severe problems of language acquisition may first be noted in primary school. In addition, problems with sound production are often identified.

Sound field systems

For educators who are having difficulty making their voices heard above the noise of the class, or who have to project their voices over some distance in large classrooms or assembly halls, or who have already experienced some vocal problems, there are systems called 'sound field systems' that will allow every learner and student in the room to hear the educator's voice. There are a number of different products on the market which involve a number of speakers placed around the room, producing an even spread of sound, making it easier for everyone to hear regardless of distance. It also allows clarity if the individual turns his/her back and speaks. The educator speaks into a microphone transmitter and his voice is projected through the speakers. However, for any sound field system to work effectively, good classroom acoustics are essential as these systems do not work well in classrooms with heavy reverberation.

As well as protecting the educator's voice, sound field systems typically benefit hearing learners and those students with hearing loss, as well as those with other auditory and learning problems. Sound field systems may help those with:

- minimal hearing loss;
- conductive hearing loss;
- fluctuating hearing loss associated with otitis media;

- unilateral hearing loss (hearing loss in one ear);
- central auditory processing disorder;
- learning disabilities;
- developmental delay;
- attention deficit;
- language delay;
- articulation disorders.

These systems are also helpful for those learning English as a second language.

Hearing checks for educators

Educators should have their hearing tested periodically because with increasing age, from 50 onwards, hearing acuity becomes less. Any diminution in hearing may be almost imperceptible from one year to the next, but the cumulative effect over many years can make it difficult for teachers to hear learners and students, or to distinguish what is being said if a number of children are talking at one time. Educators in the fields of, for example, Home Economics and Design Technology, where background noise is a feature of their teaching space, will find this particularly difficult if they have any degree of hearing loss. Hearing loss may often have the effect of making it difficult to self-monitor the loudness level of conversational speech.

Classroom acoustics

As described in Chapter 1, the structure of buildings and the materials used inside them determines their ultimate acoustic quality. Acoustic science is extremely complicated but there are, however, simple guidelines that can assist the teacher or lecturer in the use and, if necessary, the alteration or adaptation of a space.

If a space is acoustically challenging, speakers should rehearse in the space and ask for feedback on the acoustics in order to assess the required level of volume before the audience enters. Should this not be possible, a handclap will give a good indication of the degree of reverberation.

It is important to observe the size and shape of the room, the texture of the flooring, the height and shape of the ceilings, and what the ceiling surface consists of. Note the number and position of windows and other glass surfaces, the material used for window and door frames, the presence of wooden or steel beams, the furnishings (steel or wooden cupboards), chairs, and the substances used to cover walls such as notice boards, drapes, posters, curtains, pull blinds or venetian blinds, as all these will have an effect on the acoustic.

In general (and obviously all manner of combinations exist and operate differently in different spaces), low ceilings, carpeted floors, covered walls, and soft furnishings tend to 'dampen and deaden' sound and absorb the voice, making it more necessary to actively define consonants and pitch the voice appropriately, sometimes slightly higher. By contrast, hard surfaces, such as varnished timber or wooden tiles, steel-framed windows and doors, large expanses of glass and bare walls, tend to produce a bright, sharp and occasionally echoing sound. This acoustic may require a change in vocal pitch; a lower pitch may help, and a slower pace, because the reverberation of the sound can interfere with the next sound, making speech indistinct.

Modification of a difficult space is not always easy and where cost is going to be incurred professional advice should be sought. There are, however, certain inexpensive adaptations that can be trialed.

If the sound quality in the room is 'dead'
- Remove any materials such as coats (hanging on pegs) and unnecessary notice boards.
- Consider removing the carpet, provided of course that the floor surface is reasonable.
- Remove any books that are lining the walls of the room if possible.

If the sound quality in the room is 'over bright'
- Introduce screens made of an absorbent material.
- Cover the floor with a soft surface such as cork tiles, carpets, or a soft vinyl.
- Lower or pad the ceiling with absorbent material.

- Introduce more absorbent material such as drapes and bookshelves.
- Cover walls in mounted artwork.

Loss of sound over distance

When working in large spaces teachers and lecturers may encounter problems unrelated to design but related to the natural loss of sound over distance. As noted in **Chapter 1**, sound waves decrease in strength as they move away from the point at which they are initiated. To prevent the loss of the power of sound, it is important to decrease the size of the space by sectioning off the teaching area, using reflecting screens, and arranging tables and desks around the teacher to reduce the area.

When working in any space with a difficult acoustic, it is always advisable to consider the students' ability to support what they hear with information gleaned from what they see. As has already been noted, there is an element of lip-reading which underpins understanding, so visibility is essential.

Working in the open air can be challenging because of the diminution and dissipation of sound over distance; projection is compromised and leads to significant demands on the voice. Bringing groups/audience closer to the speaker or standing near a wall or on a platform can be helpful. In such spaces, whistles and megaphones can be useful to teachers and sports coaches. Public speakers should always use a public address system if one is available but should investigate ways to use them correctly and effectively. More detailed information on working outdoors can be found in **Chapter 10** while **Chapter 9** addresses the many roles of the educator using amplification.

Institution-wide vocal health in schools and universities: responsibilities and strategies

While advising educators to take responsibility for their own vocal health it is also important to consider the overall responsibility of the employer. In the case of the teacher or lecturer this would rest with head teachers/principals in schools and college governors/senior managers in Further Education, vice chancellors in Higher Education. In order to assess the degree of importance voice care was awarded in different institutions from teachers and lecturers in their first year post-qualification, Martin (2003) asked: 'Is voice care seen as important by fellow staff members?' to which the response from 94% of those questioned was 'no'. The one exception came from a teacher working in a school in which the Head Teacher had experienced voice problems herself. While wholly regrettable, there appears to be little to suggest that the same question would generate a different answer 15 years later. A 'voice care for teachers' programme (Russell *et al.*, 2007) has been initiated in the State of Victoria, Australia, by the Department of Education and Early Childhood Development, which provides a series of information sheets for principals and teachers to manage vocal health individually and collectively within a whole-school approach. It is highly commended.

Drivers for work-based change

There are, however, practical ways in which individual educators could effect change in their workplaces, to create an environment conducive to vocal health. Although it may take time for institutions to 'buy in' to change, if it prevents further vocal misuse it is always worth making a significant effort to 'beat a path' to the relevant door and drive home the importance of vocal health. In addition to changes and strategies discussed in **Chapter 4** relating to stress and anxiety, it is important to work actively with employers to make the working environment less vocally challenging, through adaptation of the physical environment and addressing physical and mental health issues affecting voice production.

Voice, as has been illustrated throughout this book, offers a particularly acute and effective gauge of mental health as well as physical health. Changes in vocal quality and delivery can indeed be some of the early indicators of mental fragility, demonstrated by lack of engagement, reduced sentence length, limited pitch range, altered intonation patterns and, if mental health issues are related to drug or alcohol addiction, a hoarse or husky vocal quality.

The following recommendations take into account institution-wide factors that can mitigate vocal misuse under the overarching categories of environmental health, physical health, and mental health.

Environmental health recommendations

- Ensure that the school buildings are kept at an even temperature.
- Ensure that windows and doors fit properly.
- Make sure that cleaning of the school is efficient and effective.
- Check that heating and ventilation systems are regularly serviced and properly maintained.
- Ensure that school grounds in cities or town centres, or near main roads, are regularly inspected for high levels of dust and debris.
- Monitor noise levels in open areas such as halls, walkways or play areas if they are near classrooms.
- If necessary, install sound baffles in open classrooms or those near to gymnasiums or practice halls.
- Provide acoustic material to reduce the level of sound reverberation in the class room.

Physical health recommendations

- Encourage a voice-free period for teachers of a minimum of 30 minutes each day.
- Make sure that there are accessible free water dispensers throughout the school or university.
- If possible provide a 'quiet' room for staff in addition to the staffroom.
- School policies should encourage staff not misuse their voice within the classroom.

- Encourage staff not to try to talk above high levels of background noise such as PA systems, music practice, or machinery in Design and Technology classes.
- Make sure teachers wear protective masks when working in dusty environments.
- Provide a humidifier for teachers working in dusty or polluted spaces.
- Discourage teachers from taking on extracurricular duties if they have a throat infection or laryngitis.
- Provide educators with portable speech amplifiers.

Occupational health and safety policies provide educators with support during times of mental fragility but for some individuals, as has been noted in detail in **Chapter 4**, mental health issues and the accompanying stress and tension will affect not only the individual's emotional state but also the ability to use the voice effectively.

The Department for Education in England announced an expansion of their school mental health initiative in 2016 (Brown, 2016) so that more schools are to benefit from working closer with mental health services. An additional pledge came from the UK government in 2017 when the then Prime Minister announced that a new approach to tackling mental health problems would start with ensuring that children and young people 'get the help and support they need and deserve'. Mental health training will be delivered by Mental Health First Aid UK to staff in a third of secondary schools in 2017, with the remaining two-thirds of secondary schools being offered the training in the following two years.

While it is hoped that the additional training will make school staff better at spotting signs of mental health problems in learners and students it is equally important that employers know how to create mentally healthy workplaces for employees. The charity, Mind, in the UK has a new initiative called 'Building on Change', which is running between 2016 and 2021 specifically to help employers engage with mental health issues among employees. They offer a 'Wellbeing Index' that employers can access in order to encourage discussion of the importance of openness regarding mental health issues.

The National Union of Teachers in the UK has produced a booklet for head teachers entitled 'Preventing Work-Related Mental Health Conditions by Tackling Stress', which offers a very positive focus on what can be done by head teachers to reduce stress among staff. Website details can be found at the end of the chapter.

Mental health recommendations

- If possible encourage adherence to working time regulations.
- Avoid setting unrealistic deadlines.
- Staff policy should encourage regular checks to see how much pressure colleagues are under.
- Encourage staff to take a statutory lunch break.
- Provide a 'safe space' where staff can go if they need to 'decompress'.
- Provide designated listening and ongoing support for staff who are struggling with mental health issues and follow through.
- Provide staff with mindfulness training for mental well-being.
- Encourage behaviour management training.
- Provide communication skills training.

Chapter Outline

- Vocal strain within the education sector
- Early warning signals and indications of vocal misuse
- Postural implications and the effect on vocal health
- Self monitoring of vocal output
- Diet/reflux
- Personal responsibilities and strategies
- Hearing and acoustics
- Institutional responsibilities
- Drivers for work based change

References and further reading

Brown J. 2016. DfE announces expansion of school mental health initiative. *Children & Young People Now*, 3 May 2016. Available at: <http://www.cypnow.co.uk/cyp/news/1157122/dfe-announces-expansion-of-school-mental-health-initiative> [Accessed August 2017].

Busch B and Jeavons P. 2016. It's time for teachers to look after their mental health – here's how. *The Guardian*, 5 June 2016. Available at: <www.theguardian.com/teacher-network/2016/jun/05/teachers-five-ways-to-boost-mental-health-mindfulness> [Accessed August 2017].

Eadicicco L. 2015. Americans check their phones 8 billion times a day. *Time Magazine*, 15 December 2015. Available at: <time.com/4147614/smartphone-usage-us-2015/> [Accessed August 2017].

Jones NS, Lannigan FJ, McMullagh M, *et al*. 1990. Acid reflux and hoarseness. *Journal of Voice* 4(4): 355–8.

Kabat-Zinn J. 2016. *Mindfulness for Beginners: Reclaiming the Present Moment and Your Life*. Boulder, CO: Sounds True.

Lemov D. 2010. *Teach Like a Champion*. San Francisco, CA: Jossey-Bass.

Mind. 2016. *Building on Change: 2016–2021*. Available at: <https://www.mind.org.uk/media/4205494/building-on-change_booklet_final_pdf_21march16.pdf> [Accessed August 2017].

National Union of Teachers (NUT) *et al*. Preventing work-related mental health conditions by tackling stress. Available at: <https://www.teachers.org.uk/files/PREVENT-WORK-REL_M_ill.pdf> [Accessed August 2017]. The NUT has already produced guidance for head teachers on 'Preventing Work-Related Mental Health Conditions by Tackling Stress', available from the health and safety section of the NUT website at: <https://www.teachers.org.uk/sites/default/files2014/preventing-work-related-mental-health-2016.pdf www.teachers.org.uk> [Accessed August 2017].

Russell A, Oates J, and Pemberton C. 2007. *Voice Care for Teachers* DVD. Available at <http://www.voicecareforteachers.com/> [Accessed April 2018].

Verdolini-Marston K, Sandage M, and Titze IR. 1994. Effect of hydration treatments on laryngeal nodules and polyps and related voice measures. *Journal of Voice* 8(1): 30–47.

Whitaker F. 2017. PM pledges free mental health training for secondary school teachers. *Schools Week*, 9 January 2017. Available at: <http://schoolsweek.co.uk/pm-pledges-free-mental-health-training-for-secondary-school-teachers/> [Accessed August 2017].

7

Communication

Professional voice users, the group to which educators belong, are, in the jargon of the day, in the 'communication business', but sometimes the skills of 'getting the message across' have either never been learned or else have been given a low priority. This is perhaps not surprising in the face of the current teacher and lecturer workload and the pre-qualification academic pressure. It is, however, one of the most essential skills for a teacher. How often are teachers and lecturers remembered for the enthusiasm and energy that they brought to the lesson rather than the content of such? Many educators are enthusiastic about their subjects but some are unable to share that enthusiasm because their communication skills are limited. This chapter explores aspects of communication and self-presentation skills that educators might find useful in their professional role.

Communication was introduced in broad terms in **Chapter 1**, when the role of voice in the communication process was discussed. In this chapter the process of communication, both verbal and non-verbal, is addressed in detail with each of its independent elements outlined below.

Language

The ability to convert ideas into words is fundamental to the communication process. There is no point in having the most wonderful appreciation of a subject without an ability to find words with which to transmit these ideas fluently and imaginatively to others, and in a form relevant to the audience.

Effective speech is the process of getting an idea from one mind to another both accurately and persuasively. There are few people who have attended lectures and not experienced the 'woolly talker' – those individuals who know exactly what they mean but are the only ones in the room who do.

This is where the choice of words, their arrangement and the way in which they are expressed, are the tools that will achieve this end most effectively. Language lives, changes, and responds to different social and cultural mores, and the fact that the English language has the capacity to change and to grow creatively by absorbing vocabulary from other cultures and countries, has made it the dynamic language that it is today. In France, where the use of grammatically correct spoken and written language is intimately connected to national identity, there was an attempt by the Academie Francaise to ban certain foreign words, mainly English and American, from advertisements and public pronouncements. The attempt was ill-conceived and subject to a certain amount of ridicule. English has always had the capacity to take and make its own vocabulary from elsewhere. This is what allows language to grow and survive in a truly pragmatic way.

So the choice of words will convey, more or less effectively, the meaning to the listener, but the way in which the words are expressed will affect the impact that the message has on the listener. Within the area of verbal communication, other parameters of speech need to be considered, namely, articulation, voice quality and vocal variety, which underpin the way that words are expressed.

Articulation

Articulation is the way in which speech sounds are produced in order to make language intelligible to the listener. The clarity of speech depends on the accuracy of the movements of the articulators: tongue, lips, jaw and teeth. The current vogue for a lack of precise articulation often leads to a loss of understanding; if what the speaker is saying is not completely understood there is a tendency for the listener to 'switch off'. Positioning plays an important role in understanding because it is often particularly difficult for learners when an educator whose articulation is not very precise stands with his back to the class, writing notes on the whiteboard and giving information at the same time. The amount of reliance on lip reading both to help and to confirm understanding has been discussed. If a speaker cannot be seen, there is often a sense that the listener needs to listen harder. To gain some appreciation of how difficult this can be, look away deliberately from a speaker and judge how much added listening effort is needed to understand them when facial expression, body posture and articulatory movements cannot be relied on to help.

There would appear to be a general perception that clear, precise articulation is somewhat outdated and decidedly unfashionable, and little value is currently placed on defined articulation. This is not to advocate a return to the rather clipped articulation of the 1940s and 1950s which black and white films so faithfully reproduce, but it is possible to be aware of articulation and to see it as a very useful tool in helping to maintain the listener's interest. With clarity of articulation there is less need for repetition and as a result, less need to use the voice unnecessarily. The muscularity of speech is never fully present if the speaker is not mentally committed to the word; on the other hand, the enthusiastic teacher with a need to share ideas rarely has a problem being understood. Only when the synchronization of thought and word occurs is language wholly energized. A return to more energized use of consonants, particularly the explosive (voiced) consonants, /b/, /d/ and /g/ and (un-voiced) /p/, /t/ and /k/, brings a dynamic to language and produces the physical and vocal movement inherent in words such as *bubble, hop, tap, bounce, kick, slap, drag,* and *giggle.*

Over-obvious manipulation of the dynamics of words is often seen as flamboyant, over-assertive or arrogant in our culture. Some individuals feel that they would be making themselves vulnerable by use of such 'over-stated' voice or that they could, or would, appear pedantic. In truth it is possible to appear all these things if articulation is pushed or unrelated to the meaning behind it, but committed meaningful speech tends to engage the breath and muscles in the most positive way and produces naturally energized language.

There is something exciting about listening to an individual who is inspired by an idea. Watching children 'hang' on the words of an effective story-teller is to know the power that language has to access the imagination of the listener. The speech of young children is full of the sounds that they hear around them – *splash*, *swoosh*, *ping*, *gurgle*, the sounds of whistles, explosions and the noise of cars, motorbikes, aeroplanes, and machinery. Of course those who read comics add words such as *Kapow!*, *Splat!*, *Zap!* and *Gadoom!* to their vocabulary, and when making these sounds they use the muscularity of speech in an uninhibited and joyous way. This playful use of the articulatory organs helps them to develop vocal and verbal muscle and imbue sound with energy that, regrettably, adults often lose. Practice, using carefully selected verse, can help to maintain the imaginative use of words, and adults too can explore their own use of language through prose and verse.

The use of the final consonant is essential in the delivery of any information and therefore critical in teaching. Conversational speech that is relaxed and delivered to one or two people does not require a deliberate weighting of consonants, but once the speech becomes public, that is to say to an audience or class, there is a need to form the consonants properly in order to aid definition and increase audibility, e.g., the final consonant in the word 'find' needs to be heard, or the word could be confused with 'fine'.

Vocal parameters

Voice, as has already been illustrated in previous chapters, works on many levels. First, it goes without saying, it makes speech audible, but it also gives definition to what is being said in many different ways, notably through changes in intonation and vocal pitch, alterations in pace, through the use of pause, by putting stress on particular syllables within words, and by emphasizing certain words in sentences. Our individual vocal identity is made up of a number of elements in a constellation of elements that provide our vocal profile, or our vocal DNA.

Intonation

Intonation, one element in this constellation, describes the way in which a specific voice alters during speech. The intonation pattern used, for example, when asking a question, is very different from the one used to express an opinion. In a situation in which a speaker feels under-confident, a questioning vocal tune may be used because it seems to produce an impression of politeness and conciliation. This 'tune' can often be heard in the voices of teachers who work with pre-primary and infant learners because it does not sound threatening or aggressive. When used inappropriately, however, it can give the impression of being uncertain and tentative. The other extreme is the continual use of the 'definite statement tune', often used by those in high status or authoritative positions and generally used by newscasters, because it is perceived as being 'the truth' and not to be questioned. Although this is a confident and assertive tune, if used inappropriately it can make learners and students, for example, feel that there is no space or opportunity to ask questions or share ideas.

Each language and dialect has an inherent 'tune' that expresses emotion and attitude. Even after a relatively short exposure to a language that is not their own, most individuals become aware of the 'tune' of the language. This then allows them, when listening to an exchange between speakers, to make an educated guess as to whether the speakers are having an argument, exchanging pleasantries or asking questions just by the way in which the individual voices are moving through the pitch range.

The benefits of understanding the intricacies of human perceptions and assumptions are obvious, particularly as educators are continually interrelating with learners, students and other members of staff on a verbal level, often with those for whom English is not their first language. Particular emphasis should be given to this vocal parameter when in an interview or an appraisal situation. More and more business and industrial courses are concentrating on the importance and power of paralinguistic skills. These are skills fundamental to the professional role but are ones that appear to receive little attention during training.

Pitch

The pitch of the voice will often carry the emotional content of speech. When an individual becomes excited or stressed, vocal pitch generally rises and the voice becomes shrill. In the same way, when frightened or very angry an individual may literally 'lose their voice' and be able only to whisper. Individuals tend to use a very low vocal pitch when they are attempting to maintain control or when they are in a situation in which they want to appear more authoritative. Despite the UK 2010 Equality Act, in practical terms discrimination against women in the work place remains and may well be expressed covertly, if not overtly. One noted reaction to this perceived inequality is the way in which women have been advized to try consciously to adopt a vocal quality that is neither too high pitched nor too light in terms of resonance, yet not so deep as to appear masculine. A lower pitch is perceived as giving more status and is thought, as a consequence, to carry more weight. Under-pitching the voice in this way, be it male or female, is not to be recommended because it can often damage the voice and limit its range, resulting in an uninteresting, limited vocal quality.

Pace and rate

Alterations in pace, the speed at which an individual speaks, greatly influence the way in which the listener interprets what is being said. If excited and enthusiastic there is a tendency to speak more quickly. Think of individuals who speak very quickly – there is a sense of urgency behind what they are saying. This device can often be used in meetings where the fast talker virtually 'steam-rollers' the meeting; the rest of the group has no chance to interrupt and scarcely time to assimilate what is being said. At the opposite end of the spectrum, if uncertain about facts or simply unsure as to what position to take on an issue, an individual may slow speech down, become hesitant and frequently introduce fillers such as 'er' and 'um', appearing to weigh up each word. A consequence of this slow delivery is that the speaker may be perceived as demonstrating uncertainty which in turn may encourage the listener to 'switch off' and disregard what is being said.

On the other hand a slow delivery may be seen as evidence of the speaker's commitment to an idea or an opinion and a sign of their confidence in expressing it. The advantage of using a fairly slow delivery rate is that it allows the speaker time to think ahead and make sure that they have complete control over what they are saying. Faster speech often does not allow the speaker to do this, and spontaneous or 'off the cuff' speech tends to be at a faster rate, although on occasions this may be the result of anxiety or stress and can result in gabbled speech. Politicians tend to use the device of slow speech, which allows them less chance of unwittingly blurting out an unreasoned opinion. To maintain the interest of the listener, however, it is important to allow the content to determine the pace of delivery, otherwise the predictability of pace becomes monotonous and unrelated to intention.

Modulation

Modulation of the voice is an important feature of communication, of how 'the message' is put across. Educators will often report that their voices lack interest or modulation: they feel that the voice is contained within a very narrow range and that it does not move in response to thought or word, and they feel that it should be 'modulated'. Modulation, however, is a word much used and often misunderstood. It suggests (erroneously) a technical changing and varying of the voice with no regard for the thought that produced it. Movement of the voice through a series of cadences without reason produces a sound just as unconnected to mind and action as a dull monotonous voice. Ideally, the voice should respond to changes in thought, these thoughts being reflected by a variety of subtle vocal changes. If, however, tension or stress levels are high it is likely that this natural delivery will be inhibited. When the individual is relaxed and at ease the voice moves effortlessly and naturally through its entire range, the movement reinforcing the intention of the language rather than distracting from it.

Pause

Pauses are often limited because it takes confidence to hold your ground, to remain silent without losing concentration, and yet crucial communication takes place in the time allowed by a pause. One piece of information should be digested before another is presented. Time constraints exert pressure to speak rapidly to get it all said so that the class can get on with the work, when often, what is being said is an absolutely essential part of the work. Pausing before important phrases, and before and after names and dates, can help listeners retain key facts. The use of the pause, rather than speaking over a noisy group, can be a valuable control mechanism.

Rhythm and energy

Rate is the speed at which an individual word or group of words is spoken. To process information effectively it is important to speak at a reasonable rate. Pace, on the other hand, can be thought of as the overall energy and rhythm of the delivery of an entire speech so that individual words can be spoken clearly and concisely, but the general pace can be driven forward energetically. This means that speech may have clarity, energy and precision as well as a sense of the 'drive' of language flowing in rhythmic cadences. The most effective way of gaining confidence in the ability to use words is to practice speaking aloud carefully selected words that trigger exciting and interesting sound patterns and images. Read aloud from the verse and prose that make up the wealth of great literature. The joy experienced when 'feeling and tasting' the vowels and consonants in the mouth is intensely rewarding. Choose passages that engender a passionate response and words that reflect personal ideas and feelings. When there is commitment behind the word, the voice reflects it naturally. More detail about the demands of reading aloud can be found in **Chapter 9.**

Vocal spontaneity

A more difficult aspect for the educator to master is the ability to make old knowledge sound new. Teachers and lecturers may have taught the same course for many years but the truly effective teacher is able to impart the information as though it was as new to them as it is to the class. When enthusiasm is natural, not pushed or forced, and the speaker uses breath freely without any postural or tension problems, most of the aspects that determine an 'interesting' voice are present. Sometimes, however, a habit of sounding monotonous has developed over a number of years and indeed, may have been with the teacher as a child or an adolescent. Habits such as vocal monotony can develop during a period of insecurity or vulnerability and frequently, when the phase passes, the habit may remain. For some adolescents, the idea of standing up in class and reading or speaking in front of their peers is terrifying; the jaw tightens and all vocal variety is suppressed. For others, a vocal quality is assumed as part of a survival strategy, such as the adolescent 'chill', 'street cred' approach, which may involve a very limited use of range. Generally these phases are natural stages of development but as with posture, the muscles often hold the pattern after the phase has passed and the voice remains limited and underdeveloped.

Gesture

Gesture provides a natural reinforcement to what is being said. French, Italian and Greek speakers are perceived as using arm and hand movements to reinforce what they are saying, whereas this is less noticeable in English and German speakers. Obviously there are exceptions to every rule but in general, gesture has cultural implications and roots. This use of gesture is referred to as 'non-verbal communication' and within this category the term 'body language' is frequently used to refer to all the means other than speech by which individuals communicate. These range from posture to small movements of the fingers, from eye contact to shaking hands. As with vocal variety, gesture should be the end result of thought processes and should stem from the desire to communicate those thoughts and ideas to the listener. Imposed gesture is quickly identified as artificial. Gesture works best when the speaker is sufficiently relaxed to integrate mind, voice and body in a total gestalt. Excessive gesture distracts from, rather than adds to, the message being conveyed.

Body language

One of the interesting things to have been discovered is how individuals who are in tune mentally, or who respect each other, tend to mirror the other's posture; this is a significant clue when looking at group dynamics. Those who are in tune are usually looking towards each other and reflecting each other's posture, whereas those who are not compatible show definite signs of defensive body posture, arms crossed, leaning away and lack of eye contact. It is perhaps appropriate for teachers and lecturers to reflect on some of the current studies available on body language that may offer strategies for them in terms of classroom management. In this way early observation of aspects of body language, which may signal disinterest, anger or depression, may be noted and contained.

Voice quality

Voice quality and vocal profile also contribute in large measure to an individual's identity and the way in which they are perceived by others. Voice quality is very influential in the impressions that individuals give and receive. The visual picture represented by the disembodied voice of the radio announcer most easily demonstrates this. This representation is partly dependent on the sound of the voice, its vocal pitch, tone and quality of resonance, partly on the accent of the speech, and partly on the content and manner of delivery.

When listeners hear an unknown voice either on the phone or out of the listener's sight they make a very definite assumption about the speaker; instinctive judgments are made about a range of attributes. These judgments can extend to the speaker's age, physical appearance including height and weight, the educational background, family background and class, status, residential area, political persuasion, level of assertiveness and intelligence. Various subtle messages, conscious and unconscious, are conveyed by the tone of the voice and it is quite possible for the words to be 'saying' one thing and the voice to be 'saying' another. A cogent example of this is where, in response to being asked how they are feeling, individuals may answer 'fine', yet it is apparent that they are not fine. Feelings of low self-esteem, tension, tiredness, sadness or boredom are all reflected in the voice.

There are certain vocal qualities that are perceived as more friendly than others. A speaker with warm 'mellow' tones seems to be perceived as someone who can be trusted, who is sincere and friendly, whereas a 'harsher', more forced voice quality can appear aggressive and threatening. The voice plays an important role in the interview situation; the advantages for the individual candidate who is able to conceal nervousness by a relaxed vocal quality and the disadvantages for another who presents with a voice that rises in pitch, seems to 'crack' and needs to be cleared constantly, are plain.

In the classroom learners and students make assumptions like everyone else. The male or female teacher who is unable to control a class often cites the voice as the cause. 'My voice isn't strong, so they don't think I mean what I say.' 'They say they can't hear me at the back of the class, so they just keep talking.' Men often find maintaining discipline easier than women and some of this can in part be attributed to their vocal quality; the lower male pitch creates a marked acoustic contrast between their vocal output and the ambient noise in the classroom.

Male teachers who have reported to the authors problems related to gaining and keeping the attention of the class have, without exception, been those with a fairly 'light' vocal quality. They reported that they had to spend a lot of time forcing their voices to produce a louder, deeper sound, and often resorted to shouting; as a consequence, they developed vocal problems. Many individuals who have problems being vocally commanding resort to shouting and often the effect of this is that, far from appearing to be in control, they are indeed perceived as having lost control. When learners and students complain that a teacher 'always sounds angry and aggressive', further questioning identifies that this is less the result of the content of what is said and more the result of the quality of vocal delivery.

Vocal texture

There are additional aspects of emphasis to be considered such as pause, pace, pitch, and stress, all of which add natural colour, texture, energy and nuance to the voice. Their use or lack of use is usually an indicator of how open or happy the individual is about engaging the breath and voice freely and responsively, rather than being the result of a lack of specific technique. Emphasis is always present when a speaker is clear about the message that he or she is conveying, just as energy is present when the speaker has a 'need' to be heard. You only have to listen to a group of enthusiasts debating a subject close to their hearts to understand this. Vocal colour is heard when a voice is well connected with the breath, has range, and is capable of pitch change. Most individuals display their true vocal colour when they laugh. Successful classroom vocal technique can create a productive environment by combining discipline and generosity. A free, generous, and unforced sound is able to develop warmth and resonance, and to convey subtle changes of thought and emotion. A voice that clearly invites the class to enter into an exchange of ideas, while at the same time being able to define the boundaries of that exchange, is an invaluable asset in a professional voice user.

Oral skills

For many people the thought of standing up and addressing a group rates as their greatest fear. The young people who are now pupils in schools will be facing the same fears in adult life, and it is sensible educational practice to develop their confidence in the area of interpersonal communication skills. If young people are given the opportunity to gain the experience and confidence needed for easy, structured and sustained public speaking, those fears need never materialize and the adults of tomorrow will be much more effective speakers.

Too often the crowded curriculum does not allow for work of this kind other than a token amount in the English syllabus. Traditionally in the UK independent fee-paying private schools have placed great emphasis on oral skills, but all children should be offered the same opportunity. Practice in oratory can be gained by reading aloud from public speeches by the great orators as these teach about effective structures. Debating societies, drama groups and involvement in reading and addressing assemblies all offer an opportunity to gain these skills. Business and industrial courses are currently teaching simple formulae for effective speech. Although they are a wonderful starting point, they are easily identified and the devices of manipulation are often obvious. Atkinson's (1984) study of oratory and politics still makes fascinating reading for anyone wanting to understand and improve the structure of formal speeches.

A new study centre 'Oracy Cambridge' at Hughes Hall, the University of Cambridge, has been working to recognize the value of good spoken communication in a diverse range of contexts – the arts, education, law, health, social care, counselling, management and other work situations – and considering how to develop a greater awareness, amongst practitioners and policy makers, of the importance of developing talk skills and of ways that this can be pursued in practice. An initiative between the English Speaking Union and School 21 (oracynetwork.org) has published a collection of essays entitled 'Speaking Frankly' by teachers, academics and educational thinkers on the importance of oracy in education, and their drive to renew interest in oracy is to be commended; the work at School 21 and other schools throughout the UK, who are using their resources and philosophy, have produced demonstrable and very promising results. **Chapter 8** offers ideas for developing oracy skills in the classroom.

Attention skills

Small children often have poorly developed listening and attention skills; they may also have problems of auditory immaturity. Infant and elementary school teaching is often through the auditory channel. In order to reduce vocal effort teachers should encourage children to look and listen for signals that are not vocal.

It is useful to begin each term and half term with a refresher session where the teacher recaps on the procedures involved in listening and looking, such as:

- Highlighting the importance of the child's active involvement in this process.
- Reminding them of the need to remember to 'look and listen' to the teacher throughout the day, reinforcing the 'good listening', 'good looking', 'good sitting'.
- Using an alternative non-vocal approach to ask for the class's atten-

tion, such as a large cardboard hand with 'Stop' written on it which can be raised to indicate that the class must be quiet and await instructions; cardboard traffic lights on a stick with the stoplight painted a vivid red can be used as well.

- Encouraging children to keep a watchful eye on the teacher as this is good for working on visual attention and developing 'good looking' skills.
- Using cymbals and drums to signal silence: when the sound is heard the class must stop talking and be quiet.
- Employing the use of a 'round robin' message that follows a well designated pathway. The teacher gives her request to Child A, who is nearby; Child A passes on the message to Child B, and so on around the class. Choose a specific brief instruction such as 'Be quiet' or 'Put your books away and stand in line'.

Explaining

It is self evident that despite the increased use of information technology, the teacher will spend most of the working day talking, either in small group situations with individual children or, as in most secondary school classrooms or in further or higher education lecture rooms, as a public performance. Not all this time is, however, spent in simple transmission. Studies by Martin (2003) noted that teachers reported that on average they spent 60% of each lesson talking. Ogunleye (2002) reported an even greater proportion of lesson time: 80% spent in teacher talk across further education colleges, with student talk accounting for 17.3% and silence or non-event, for 2% of the lesson.

Given these findings it is not surprising that educators report vocal fatigue but additionally report that a great deal of contact time is spent in re-explaining information that has already been given to learners and students. This is not only vocally tiring and frustrating but can be unprofitable. If the quality of the explanation is poor, the time is spent ineffectually. A review of the literature suggests that good explanations are not only clearly structured but also interesting.

Explanation: strategies and skills

Explaining can be described as a mixture of strategies and skills which need to be mastered if explanations are going to be effective. Teachers, lecturers and trainers, and indeed anyone who is in the explanation business, needs to remember this. Brown's (1986) suggestions for explanation effectiveness still remain highly relevant today. He suggested that topics should be analysed into main parts and:

- links should be established between these parts;
- the characteristics of the learner must be accounted for when adapting plans; and
- if there are any rules involved in the explanation they should be defined.

Brown also suggests that those giving the explanation must have certain basic skills, such as:

- clarity and fluency;
- emphasis and interest;
- use of examples; and
- organiazation and feedback.

It can therefore be seen that synergy of what is said, how it is said and the social relationship in which the speech is embedded, is critical; an articulate teacher is likely to be judged an effective teacher.

When Brown asked students for feedback regarding their main dissatisfaction with teachers and lecturers their responses related to the teachers' and lecturers'

- failure to emphasize main points;
- failure to pitch at an appropriate level;
- inaudibility;
- incoherence; and
- reading aloud from notes.

Clarity and fluency can be achieved through defining new terms, use of explicit language and avoiding vagueness. Emphasis and interest can be achieved by variations in gesture, use of media and materials, use of voice and pauses and repetition, paraphrasing or verbal cueing.

Examples, when used, should be of sufficient quantity, clear, appropriate and concrete and, where applicable, positive and negative. The organization of the lecture, lesson or explanation should be in a logical and clear sequence with the use of link words and phrases. Feedback to the listener should provide opportunities for questions and there should be an assessment of what the listener has understood of the main idea. In addition, the individual giving the explanation should seek to understand the attitudes and values of those to whom they are speaking.

Many of the above issues that cause student dissatisfaction are easy to remedy and could make a considerable difference to class response. Recent studies by John Hattie (*The Educators*, 2015) suggest that the quality of the teachers' interest and passion for their subjects has the most effect on student learning. Even if the subject is not one that the students are specifically interested in, the students report that the passion of the teacher makes learning fun and makes them good at their subject.

Presentation

The dynamics of the workplace are often affected for good or ill by something as simple as the clothes that an individual is wearing, his/her posture, voice quality and national and/or regional accent. All these aspects form part of the communication process – the way in which individuals interact with one another in a social context. These paralinguistic features will determine how an individual is judged by those with whom they come into contact and, like it or not, these value judgments, often the product of prejudice, are deeply entrenched and difficult to alter once they have been made. Within the teaching profession, value judgments made of educators by learners or students will critically affect the relationship between them and influence, for better or worse, the dynamic within the classroom. The same is true, of course, among fellow professionals in whatever occupation. Students are just as likely to be victims of these judgments. Knowledge by teachers of these paralinguistic features may alleviate judgments of this kind.

Accent and dialect

Recognition should also be given to the fact that accent and dialect are often the criteria on which initial impressions are formed. Intrinsically, accents carry certain intonation patterns, which according to the listener's individual perception, may appear to have more or less musical quality and therefore acceptability, depending on their individual preference. Musicality, however, has a hidden cost; individuals with a musical accent are sometimes perceived as lacking authority. The inflection pattern, which gives the more musical sound, can at times be falsely interpreted as questioning and uncertain.

Discussion about accents and the assumptions that are made about accents, well documented by Honey in 1989, is still live almost three decades later and should be challenged in the classroom, otherwise change will never occur. Nevertheless, newly qualified teachers with a specific regional accent should be aware that accent is, for some, an emotive issue. A teacher with a non-local accent may be positively perceived or conversely, the difference may be the basis for ridicule, particularly from adolescent learners or students. Younger children seem much more generous, but adolescents often take their attitudes from the media which does nothing to break the stereotypical assumptions of regional accent but rather, to reinforce them. The accent with which an individual speaks is usually the one spoken in the area in which they were raised and the one used by their primary carer. Today, however, so many family units move from one area to another that many children have parents with different accents or different first languages. Children who move in their early years generally adopt the accent of their peer groups in an effort to conform and be accepted. This transition from one accent to another happens very quickly in some children, in a matter of a few weeks.

By the middle teens accent is less likely to alter; adults seldom change their accents dramatically although most individuals are 'vocal chameleons',

slightly adapting their speech according to changing situations – the phenomenon of the 'telephone voice' is well recognized. Adults, however, rarely
make a conscious decision to change their accents unless for very specific
political or socio-cultural reasons. A teacher from Leicester, whose accent is
completely 'London', provides a useful example here. This teacher had taught
in south-east London for many years, during which time he had consciously
allowed his accent to change because he felt that it was easier for the class to
relate to him. This is not a common occurrence; the richness of regional and
national accents should enrich the life of the classroom and teachers should
not feel a need to eradicate or seek to eradicate their accent. Nevertheless,
people's accents may be devalued. A Jamaican teacher, known to the authors,
provides an illustration of this. The teacher, in an attempt consciously to alter
her accent, was misusing her voice. Her written comment after attending a
voice care and development training course was as follows: 'felt valued as a
Jamaican, I wasn't put down. Hurrah!' Whether this teacher had been 'put
down' in the past because of her accent was not known, but certainly she felt
that a lack of respect for her nationality was inextricably linked to her accent,
and the perception other people had of it and hence of her. This small cameo
illustrates the considerable significance placed on accent.

Educators should attempt to ensure clarity and vocal spontaneity, whatever their accent, and promote tolerance in children by encouraging them to
talk about the diversity of speech in the institution, community and region.
When children understand the reason for differences they cease to mock
them. Should a teacher feel that his accent is an issue in the teaching arena
it is possible to initiate an open discussion about accent and dialect so that
different accents within the class are also accepted positively. Many learners
and students will have parents who speak with another accent and who may
speak differently from others in the class. Conurbations are more likely to
have a wide variety of accents. Distinctions should be made between clarity
and accent so that students can be offered the opportunity to develop a wide
vocabulary, eloquence, and a joy in communicating verbally.

Vocal perceptions and impressions

What are the factors that determine first or initial impressions? Substantial research has affirmed the importance of first impressions while exploring a variety of factors that contribute to their formation. For example, a 2009 study in *Personality and Social Psychology Bulletin* found that factors ranging from clothing style to posture play a role in how impressions are formed. A study in the April 2011 issue of *Social Influence* found, for example, that even a limp handshake may influence personal judgments as it may make one appear overly passive.

A major component of a 'first impression' is visual, what is seen: the person's appearance, posture, body language, facial expression, eye contact. What is heard, namely the voice quality, the pitch of the voice, the pace and use of pause, the clarity of speech and the accent that the person has, determines the auditory component of an initial impression, whereas the words that are said are initially very low on the list. It may seem almost unbelievable that through what appears to be a rather arbitrary set of criteria, decisions are made which will affect future relationships, but that in fact is what appears to happen. The validity of this form of judgment lies in the fact that most people when asked how often they have altered their first impression of someone will respond 'rarely'.

A major barrier to interpersonal communication lies in an individual's natural tendency to judge – to approve or disapprove of – the statements of the other person. Statements do not need to be verbal; as has been said earlier, statements are made by an individual's choice of clothes, hairstyle, facial expression and body language. So how does this process work?

When forming an impression of other people, individuals are influenced by a set of beliefs and values, known in psychology as the false-consensus effect, or false-consensus bias, in which they overestimate the extent to which their opinions, beliefs, preferences, values, and habits are normal and typical of those of others, and their belief that other people have similar beliefs. This cognitive bias tends to lead to the perception of a consensus that does not exist, a 'false consensus'.

This false consensus is significant because it increases self-esteem (over-confidence effect). It is derived from a desire to conform and be liked by others in a social environment. This bias is especially prevalent in group settings where one thinks the collective opinion of the group matches that of the larger population. Since the members of a group reach a consensus and rarely encounter those who dispute it, they tend to believe that everybody thinks the same way. The false-consensus effect is not restricted to cases where people believe that their values are shared by the majority, but it still manifests as an over-estimation of the extent of their belief. When these values and beliefs are extreme, objective assessment becomes impossible. Colour prejudice is a particularly evident and malicious example of this, as are sexual, gender, religious and age prejudice. In forming relationships with other people, individuals want to have their own ideas and beliefs reflected, the well recognized tendency for individuals to 'like people like themselves'. (Details of useful websites can be found at the end of this chapter.)

Educators, similarly, need to recognize that learners and parents, students, staff members and school visitors make instinctive judgments at the beginning of every school year, and past students may reflect on their judgments of a particular teacher. 'You've got Mrs Fisher this year. Oh goodness, she is so boring and it is really difficult to hear her.' Consequently, the received wisdom is that Mrs Fisher is boring and inaudible, even if this was a value judgment made by a student several years before.

It is also important to recognize that the tendency to evaluate is very much heightened in those situations where feelings and emotions are deeply involved. The stronger the feelings, the more likely it is that there will be no middle ground; there will be two ideas, two feelings, and two judgments, all missing each other. For teachers, lecturers and trainers this situation is predictable; the students are anxious about moving into a new class, and the teacher is equally anxious about the new students. What will the class be like? Will there be problems of discipline? An incorrect assumption early on in a relationship can determine the ongoing communication, often with critical results. After all, there are few professions where such an intimate relationship exists over such an extended period as that between teachers, lecturers and trainers and their learners and students.

Given the need to maximize the opportunity to communicate effectively, how can this be achieved? There are several well recognized communication facilitators that can be applied in any situation, as discussed below.

Facilitating communication

Positioning

How an individual is positioned in relation to another person or persons is very important; each position 'says' something. It is not always possible to choose where to sit, but the position can affect the interaction that takes place in significant and predictable ways. There is a tendency to sit opposite a competitor; this obviously has much to do with a desire and a need to be in a position to monitor the other person's movements. In education there is very little choice; positioning is fairly well prescribed by the number of pupils and the need to view the whiteboard, overheads, PowerPoint or audiovisual aids. In primary school this is easier; more teaching can be undertaken in a round-table setting which also encourages a more participative atmosphere, even if a noisier one. Wherever possible teachers should try to vary the placement of desks and encourage more participative positions.

When considering interview situations, e.g., when visiting the doctor or someone in authority, this 'opposite position' appears to be the preferred position, although more doctors are introducing a diagonal position vis-à-vis the patient, which is similar to that of an 'interview' situation. Sitting or standing alongside another individual is the recognized co-operative position, but that is more rarely seen in formal situations. Needless to say, this would be most difficult for teachers to achieve in junior or secondary schools, but it could be achieved in small group tutorials or discussion groups and is certainly to be recommended.

If learners are seated so that they can see the teacher's face when instructions are given it will greatly help understanding and reduce the vocal effort and volume required by the teacher. It is important for male teachers to remember that moustaches and beards make lip reading more difficult so they will need to compensate by articulating clearly. When working in acoustically difficult spaces, children should be grouped around the teacher, thereby lessening the need for excessive volume.

Distance

Distance from another person or group of people would not at first sight appear to be an important aspect of communication, but it has been recognized as having a considerable effect. Studies have highlighted appropriate distances for specific communication situations. From nought to half a metre is an appropriate distance for intimate social situations, half a metre to one and a half metres for personal situations, talking to good friends or colleagues for example, whereas social/consultative situations require a distance of one and a half to three metres to be maintained between people. For public situations more than three and a half metres between speaker and audience is appropriate. This suggests that for many teachers and lecturers there is a positioning mismatch within the classroom environment. For those pupils sitting at the front of the class, they and the teacher relate at a 'personal' distance, whereas for those further back, the relationship is one of a 'social/consultative' distance. Educators should be aware of this and attempt to compensate for it by perhaps addressing more comments to the back of the class, spending more time making eye contact with those at the back of the class, looking at their posture in relationship to those at the back, and indeed deliberately moving around the class so that they achieve a mix of 'personal' and 'social consultative' positioning with all learners and/or students.

Positive teaching styles

Arrangement of the class or lecture room should allow for the free movement of both pupils and staff. It should allow the teacher or lecturer to stand beside or behind each pupil or student when teaching and make verbal, visual or physical contact with each child. Anecdotally, teachers report that they can modify 'bad' behaviour by walking up to the child or student and, putting a hand firmly on their shoulder, exerting gentle pressure and saying nothing. 'A gentle hand on the shoulder' may work but members of the teaching profession will be very aware of the guidelines regarding physical contact with pupils and students, so this is an approach that needs to be used with care and confidence, and discussed in staff meetings in order to avoid any potential misunderstanding of intent. It is obviously inadvisable to use any form of pressure that could be interpreted as pushing, jostling, threatening or sexual in any way.

In attempting to maintain order in class, teachers report that their greatest resource is their ability to observe and assess the mood of the class and to remain vigilant without becoming reactive to the class's manipulation. Most teachers find that objective observation allows them to change the class's behaviour without losing respect and co-operation. When teachers were questioned, most reported that they found talking, deliberate hindering, idleness, and pupils being out of their seats the most annoying aspects of class behaviour, specifically because it is these behaviours that considerably reduce teaching time. Students and learners are quick to observe vulnerability and disruptive elements among the student population will inevitably try to capitalize on this.

Positive reinforcement

'Nagging' is deeply wearying for educators, may lead to accusations of bullying and seldom changes the student's behaviour; rather, it may simply inflame a difficult situation and create a rather fruitless and negative atmosphere within the classroom. Educators recognize their own tendency to 'nag' but report that it has often been difficult to find alternative effective responses.

It is obviously important to minimize negative responses, maximize positive responses, and reinforce good behaviour. When the negative response is used sparingly, its effectiveness is considerable; when used constantly the effectiveness is minimized. Teachers and lecturers admitted, when questioned, that their reinforcement of positive attitudes to academic standards far outweighed their positive attitudes to social behaviour. It is often common to comment on lack of effort rather than praise pupils who continue to do what they are told without causing any trouble. Positive reinforcement should be used with honesty so that children see it as genuine and well deserved; they quickly see through 'phoney' praise and this therefore invalidates real effort.

Educators will be very aware of the importance of approval and disapproval to learners and students, but in the often-frenetic atmosphere of the classroom it is sometimes difficult not to 'reserve' approval for really major effort and focus more on instances of wrong-doing.

Negotiation skills

A major cause of stress develops as a result of poor negotiation within the classroom setting or the staffroom. A great deal of tension can be defused by the application of effective negotiation strategies. A major cause of adolescent rebellion and staff discontent comes about through the frustration that results when individuals find themselves in 'no win' situations. The old style authoritarian approach places people in the position of feeling that if one person wins, the other loses. Negotiations that work to find 'win/win' agreements (where both sides feel that they have won) rather than 'win/lose' situations leave everyone happy, productive and co-operative as a result.

Young people who, quite rightly, are being taught to 'know their rights' often have difficulty understanding that other people also have the same rights, problems and needs. On the one hand they are told to 'be assertive' and 'learn to say no' but on the other, they are accused of being 'self-centred' and 'stubborn'. Assertiveness, when it does not take the needs of others into consideration, becomes a form of bullying. It takes maturity to be able to find the workable solution to problems that seem irresolvable. Most adolescents have a highly developed sense of justice and can therefore easily relate to the fairness of the 'win/win' negotiation. To bring about such an agreement it is necessary to break through the deadlock that is the result of individuals being unwilling to accept the other person's point of view. Concessions often need to be made and these should be made on both sides. When one party is expected to concede too much without due recognition and discussion of their needs, the result is a breakdown in communication, feelings of resentment and a withdrawal of goodwill. Such situations benefit neither party and serve only to increase general stress levels. A potentially difficult situation requiring sensitive negotiation is that of parents' evening where both the child and parent/carer may be present.

Negotiation skills can be learned from books or better still by the organization of a staff development or in-service workshop. The information gleaned from such training can be passed on to students by the application of strategies to the classroom situation and formally within the oral element of the English class. Many schools have Personal and Social Skills classes, and these skills could be usefully shared in such an arena. Schools are also responsible for the Personal Social Health and Economic Education (PSHE) programme for ages 5 to 18, and this incorporates many aspects of personal and social development, emotional literacy, emotional intelligence, social and emotional competence and social, emotional and behavioural skills. The Social and Emotional Aspects of Learning (SEAL) initiative is available to all primary schools in England and funding is given to local authorities to provide training and support to primary schools to implement and embed SEAL (from 3 to 11 years). These initiatives are just two examples where oral skills are of considerable importance and where those with limited oral skills may be impoverished.

Schools with specific problems such as bullying and racism can apply the principles of 'win/win' negotiation in order to bring about understanding and reconciliation. The teacher who is able to apply the principles of fair negotiation to a difficult discipline problem could find that not only has the specific problem been solved but also, the change in tactics alters the atmosphere of the classroom for the better and indeed, influences the group culture within the school. While a confrontational situation exists there will be no winners and the teacher's voice will suffer.

For many teachers, the most difficult time to maintain discipline is as the children come in and go out of the classroom. Keeping the children outside the door for a little longer and giving instructions at that time is worthwhile, e.g., 'go in quietly, sit at your desk and get out your books' is more effective than trying to give instructions as children come into the classroom, when the level of noise is much higher and teachers have to fight against this to make themselves heard.

Teachers questioned for a UK television programme were very aware of the 'good day/bad day syndrome' and were able to offer opinions as to why these occur. There was agreement that negative responses tended to occur when teachers were ill-prepared for the class, unsure of their material, or under external and personal stress. Teachers recognized that their moods were often dictated by a wide variety of situations, but it was particularly important to allow sufficient recovery time from a previous situation. If, for example, there was a lack of recovery time from the effect of family tensions, a difficult journey to school, an unpleasant incident in the previous lesson or an early morning staffroom rush, this could impinge on the entire school day. It is important to remember to try to break this type of pattern, or at least to be aware of situations that can precipitate it, and if possible, to make changes to allow more time to recover. Educators may recognize that it is important to delegate activities, to admit to needing help and to try to use all possible means of reducing areas of tension within their working environment, but finding a way of achieving this is very difficult.

Dealing with the voice of doubt

Educators, like actors, often have to contend with niggling doubts about their own ability. This is especially difficult when a disruptive class undermines their status and confidence. Most teachers admit to thoughts such as 'I can't do this', 'I can't control this group', 'The class thinks I'm a walk over', 'This class is going so badly. It must be my fault'; 'I should have prepared this better'. This 'self-speak' can be as undermining and hurtful as if it were being said by an examiner or a colleague. It is also difficult to control once it has started and must be challenged.

Many teachers, lecturers, and trainers, speak about walking into a room, whether this be a classroom, lecture hall, or training room, feeling that they have lost the battle before they have even started. It is important to notice what such an attitude does to the body and how it subsequently affects the breath and therefore vocal use. Consider for a moment the posture of defeat and that of victory as well as the postures for wellbeing and depression. In defeat the shoulders round forward, the spine slumps, the head comes down and the eye level drops. All this leads to a reduced space between the hips and ribs and results in diminished breath capacity. Feeling confident and positive lengthens the spine, opens out the chest. The weight is balanced and the head is poised on the top of the spine, allowing the eye level to lift and open up peripherally. There is also considerable space between the hips and lower ribs allowing for breath to be full and low. There are of course dangers in striding arrogantly into a situation because learners and students may 'read' this as a message of physical aggression, so it is important always to be aware of the subtext of the language of the posture.

How does the teacher develop a positive 'self-speak'? The first step in doing this is to acknowledge that negative self-programming exists. Educational consultant, Mary Johnson, illustrates this concept by recounting how teachers were asked to address a class while negative suggestions were whispered in their ear. The teachers reported on how negative this made them feel. The exercise was repeated with affirmative comments which produced positive, confidence-building reactions. Generally, teachers were able to relate to this exercise and to acknowledge that they often undermine themselves unnecessarily. This was particularly likely when morale was low, or they had been experiencing difficulties on a regular basis, so they anticipated failure before they even encountered it. It is important to look beyond the difficult situation to the teacher's desire and commitment to teach and enhance the lives of young people. By reminding themselves of their aspirations and learning to excuse the occasional badly handled situation, it becomes easier to re-discover the joys of teaching. Carrying demoralizing thinking and low self-esteem from difficult situations into new challenges can only be limiting and ultimately damaging.

It is worth remembering that good communication skills indicate that speakers not only respect their audience, but also value themselves.

Above all teachers should be supported in working on their own voices. The teacher who is aware of the role that their voice plays in communication is clearly advantaged. Kathy, an experienced teacher and trainer, explains her relationship to her voice and her craft:

> How I sound, whether I am shrieking and pushing the voice or sounding dull and monotonous, will affect the students at an unconscious level. I need to be able to read all the clues: If I am breathy it may be that I am too reliant on what others are thinking. If I am not finishing my words this has something to do with a lack of trust in what I am saying.
>
> If my pitch is restricted I am not playful. Pitch is released by a sense of joy and diminished by a lack of it. Teachers in the primary school often tend to have more playfulness in their voices than the teachers in the secondary schools. If I try to control through a rigid, inflexible pitch it eliminates a sense of fun and a sense of freedom. When my body is relaxed enough to allow a free and varied use of pitch, it also has open resonating spaces so my voice has resonance.
>
> Control is seen as such a highly desirable thing in the classroom and so sometimes I control in the wrong way and the consonants are held on to and the vowels are lost. This leads to the control being there in the voice but the feeling and empathy is not. Discipline is necessary but in our 'culture of control' we often forget to share the control with the children. If I share the control with them they are in control of their learning.
>
> If we can read these things in ourselves, we can read our students better. Teaching is hard, and I have learned that you need to have access to all of yourself and if your voice is locked it means that all of you is not accessible. The teacher has to be so many

things to the class and the current role is often conveyed by the voice, both by non-verbal language and by the tonal quality and music of the voice.

Finding help

Many education authorities engage expert advisers who are available to support educators. Consultant Mary Johnson offers an example of a typical case study illustrating how changes in classroom strategies, both practical and attitudinal, can prove helpful:

> When I am asked to give support to teachers in difficulty, I usually observe the teacher in the classroom and then consult with subject specialists, so that we can offer the teacher practical strategies in order to overcome the particular challenges. An example of this was a young teacher I was asked to help whose subject was science. She was struggling to make herself heard in the classroom and there were other aspects of her teaching practice that needed support and development. She hadn't yet lost her voice, but she lacked vocal command and, sometimes, was simply inaudible.
>
> The year 8 class was a small but lively one. There were several things about the set-up of the classroom that immediately put her at a disadvantage. The tables were fixed, the space was large and the 15 students were spread throughout the lab behind these imposing tables. This physical separation meant that there was little cohesion or sense of joint enterprise. The importance of the lesson and the possibilities for communication were immediately undermined.
>
> The students talked or sometimes called to one another. The teacher talked over them and they talked over her. Her anxiety rose and affected her breathing, making it shallower. In most situations like this the teacher's 'self-talk', what she is saying inwardly and often unconsciously to herself, turns negative and

further increases her anxiety. As this teacher's breathing became shallower, giving less and less support to her voice, she became shriller. She tried not to shout, but as her frustration grew she began to shriek at the class. Her natural musical quality flattened out and her voice became strained and inflexible.

She was given help with the physical arrangement of the classroom. This was essential not only so that the students were involved in the lesson but also so that she could speak less. She realized that she must never speak over the class: not only did this produce more vocal strain but they simply wouldn't be listening. She learned how to get their attention without speaking.

She was also given support in creating more varied and inclusive lessons. These strategies included using a wider range of learning styles with more practical work, some individual learning packages and increased paired work. All of this together with the alteration in the classroom set-up and her vocal changes greatly improved the whole learning experience. Her confidence increased and she enjoyed her working life more.

There were, however, personal issues that needed to be addressed as well. Her home life was quite stressful: she had two young children and was taking responsibility for most of the domestic chores. This meant she spent hardly any time on herself, on relaxation and personal enrichment. I had noticed that her natural and unstressed vocal quality was musical and discovered that she had been a singer. I encouraged her to find time to start singing again as a way of investing in herself, developing her confidence and reclaiming the musicality of her voice.

We need to make the 'soft skills' central to education and educators. We need to support teachers in developing their own expressiveness so that they become more dynamic and confident in the classroom. Self-esteem and relationship dynamics and the effective use of voice, movement and space are among the skills that are often neglected in teacher training. Yet these are central to the quality of the learning experience. We need to pay them much more attention.

Chapter outline

- Language
- Articulation
- Vocal parameters
- Aspects of modulation
- Oral skills
- Attention skills
- Explaining
- Presentation
- Accent and dialect
- Vocal perception and impressions
- Facilitating communication
- Negotiation skills
- Dealing with the voice of doubt

References and further reading

Atkinson M. 1984. *Our Masters' Voices*. London: Routledge.

Bernieri F and Petty KN. 2011. The influence of handshakes on first impression accuracy. *Social Influence* 6: 78–87.

Brown GA. 1986. Explaining. In: Hargie O (ed.) *A Handbook of Communication Skills*. London: Croom Helm.

Fabrigar LR and Krosnick JA. 1995. Attitude importance and the false consensus effect. *Personality and Social Psychology Bulletin* 21(5): 468–79. Available at: <https://pprg.stanford.edu/wp-content/uploads/1995-Attitude-importance-and-the-false-consensus-effect.pdf> [accessed August 2017].

Government Equalities Office. 2013. *Equality Act 2010: Guidance.* Available at: <https://www.gov.uk/guidance/equality-act-2010-guidance> [Accessed August 2017].

Hattie J. 2014. *The Educators,* BBC Radio 4. Broadcast on 25 August, 2014. Available at: <http://www.bbc.co.uk/programmes/b04dmxwl> [Accessed August 2017].

Honey J. 1989. *Does Accent Matter?* London: Faber and Faber.

Mugglestone L. 2003. *Speaking Proper* (2nd edn). Oxford and New York, NY: Oxford University Press.

Naumann LP, Vazire S, Rentfrow PJ, and Gosling SD. 2009. Personality judgments based on physical appearance. *Personality & Social Psychology Bulletin* 35(12): 1661–71.

Ogunleye J. 2002. An investigation of curriculum arrangements conducive to fostering creativity in post-compulsory education and training institutions. PhD thesis, University of Greenwich, London.

Oracy Cambridge: *The Hughes Hall Centre for Effective Spoken Communication.* Available at: <http://oracycambridge.org> [Accessed August 2017].

Oracy Network. Available at: <http://www.esu.org/our-network/oracy-network> [Accessed August 2017].

Raki T, Steffens MC, and Mummendey A. 2011. When it matters how you pronounce it: The influence of regional accents on job interview outcome. *British Journal of Psychology* 102: 868–83.

Tannen D. 1998. *The Argument Culture.* London: Virago Press.

Tannen D. 1992. *You Just Don't Understand.* London: Virago Press.

Wells JC. 1982. *Accents of English.* Cambridge: Cambridge University Press.

Williams A and Kerswill P. 1999. Dialect levelling: change and continuity in Milton Keynes, Reading and Hull. In: Foulkes P and Docherty G (eds.) *Urban Voices.* London and New York, NY: Routledge.

8

Words in the teaching environment

In the classroom, most of the communication between teacher and student is word based. Anecdotal reports suggest that many teachers feel that their vocal problems arise from the difficulty that they have in finding and using words effectively. Voice production is most effective when what is being said is important to the speaker and subsequently, stimulating to the listener. Teachers are often conscious that their difficulties began as a result of a lack of focus on oral skills in their own education and training, and feel that they would like to offer a richer spoken language environment to their students. It would seem appropriate therefore to use this chapter to offer suggestions for raising the vocal and verbal profile of the classroom.

Vocal persona

No matter how dedicated a teacher is, his/her success will depend upon more than dedication, passion and knowledge. It will require the ability to project a persona that engages, inspires and commands authority and respect.

The moment teachers enter a room they bring with them a persona. Assumptions are made by the students immediately on that first impression. Posture, status and confidence, clothing, general attitude, demeanour, the way in which they use and structure language and above all, their vocal delivery, all provoke a response in the students from which they form a perception of the teacher. These perceptions may be incorrect: if the voice used is strident it might suggest an aggressive quality; if posture is slumped it might suggest a lack of confidence; or if eye contact is not made, it might suggest insincerity or dis-engagement with the group. None of these may be the case but all could be interpreted negatively. While perceptions can be inaccurate, once established they can be difficult to change.

Some educators suggest adopting a 'mask' or persona through which a teacher's passion for the work can shine while preserving or shielding personal integrity; others feel the teacher should allow personal beliefs and authenticity to be exposed.

What is important is that teachers and lecturers are aware of how body language and vocal tone and can be interpreted. This is best done by observation of others and developing knowledge of one's own habitual voice and body use. Awareness of personal movement patterns and physical and vocal idiosyncrasies can be difficult to perceive and analyse, so a video recording and feedback from an objective colleague is worth considering.

Humans are complex and multi-faceted and we respond in a variety of ways depending on where and who we are. We use different body language and vocabulary depending on who is being addressed and the formality of the situation. This does not suggest we are insincere or false but that our emotional intelligence determines the way in which we adjust our personas when responding to a given situation, leading to an emphasis of different aspects of our personalities. It also means that there is an element of choice in our responses and that we, like actors, can adapt and perform in a way that is appropriate to the learning environment, the subject matter and the age of the group.

There is some debate as to how much 'acting' is acceptable and whether or not teachers should assume false confidence by wearing a 'mask', as by doing so they could lose their authenticity. In *The Elements of Teaching* (Banner and Cannon, 1997) it is suggested that "a trap young teachers often fall into is that of assuming 'teaching personalities' that are not their own. Such teachers are like unconscious actors; they are playing roles based, often unknowingly on the favourite school teachers or college mentors of their own youth".

In his excellent Princeton University blog *Academic Librarian* (December 2008), lecturer Wayne Bivens-Tatum questions whether assuming a persona should always be considered a trap. He writes of his early teaching experience: 'I could no more have been myself in front of those 18-year-olds then I could have plausibly played the greybeard. Still, based upon readings at the time on teaching persona, I did deliberately fashion one for the class, and it was indeed based upon a specific professor I'd had in college, which is not to say that it wasn't also me'. Bivens-Tatum goes on to say that as he became a more confident teacher his 'classroom persona' blended more closely with his own. Without the fear of losing control and with more confidence he was able to reveal more of himself. (Details of the blog can be found at the end of this chapter.)

The effects of technology

The teacher and lecturer use words, either spoken or written, in almost every activity that they undertake. Language and its delivery underpin the way that knowledge is imparted. The modern approach to the process of education is a two-way exchange of ideas between teacher and student and therefore depends on the ability of both to participate effectively. Society, however, is moving increasingly towards a use of technology that does not always encourage interactive verbal skills. Although the ability of the young to use technology is essential, it is imperative that the balance is redressed by the equivalent development of speech and language skills.

Schools, colleges, and universities are becoming more dependent on technology as a method of teaching. It is seen as a way of releasing teachers from contact time and often provides an effective method of instruction for subjects such as (ironically) languages. The growth of e-learning is increasingly used to provide students with a teaching medium that may be conducted entirely on their own – interaction is limited to that of the computer screen. Lecturers often use PowerPoint presentations supported by handouts when teaching large groups, which can limit discussion. Others are taught by on-line modules with feedback given electronically.

Today's children are used to interacting with computer technology and obtain both entertainment and information from screens. Many have their own smart-phones and tablets. Although the educational value of television and other forms of media cannot be under-estimated, the result of young schoolchildren spending time as passive viewers rather than active doers has reduced reading time and has led to an erosion of the broad range of expression available to children. Many children entering school are unable to use language to communicate; they do not have sufficient experience of conversation at home, and nursery and primary teachers are expressing concern about communication skills in the early years. It cannot be taken for granted that children are exposed to the level of conversation they require in order for them to thrive in the education system. An article by Alison Shepherd in the *Times Educational Supplement* (2005) remains pertinent: 'Surveys show that the more young children are talked to the better they express themselves and the greater their achievements in later life. Yet foundation stage teachers complain that the language skills of each fresh intake of children are deteriorating'. Shepherd quotes literacy consultant, Sue Palmer, who says: 'It [language] underpins learning: you cannot learn unless you can express and explore what is in front of you'. In her book *Toxic Childhood* (2007) Palmer highlights the problem: '4- and 5-year-olds were coming to school with poorer language skills than ever before; they were not arriving with the repertoire of nursery rhymes and songs little ones used to know ...'.

Some children and young adults are prevented from accessing the curriculum fully because they are unable to communicate effectively. Considerable amounts of Government funding have been and are being awarded to Sure Start schemes in areas of social deprivation in order to give specialized communication skills training to help to prepare children for the educational environment (details of the website can be found at the end of this chapter). Better education for parents as to the need to develop early language skills in their children is required. Unfortunately, with many parents needing to return to work as soon as possible, the regular contact many pre-school children have is either not one to one, or is sometimes from a nanny or other care giver who speaks English as a second language and cannot be expected to know traditional English nursery rhymes and stories. Care givers should be encouraged to speak their own rhymes and sing their own traditional songs to children, thus exposing them to other language structure, sound, and rhythm. There are compact disc recordings of age-appropriate music that can be played and sung along to.

The problem is not limited to early years and older children, similarly, may display limited language skills; teachers increasingly report that their students are using language mechanically and automatically, that they are using words without thought. For this reason, many teachers express a keen interest in returning to the teaching of oral skills that provide the opportunity to enjoy words and foster a delight in the speaking of well ordered and expressive language; skills that have been 'side-lined' by the crowded curriculum. It is important to be clear that the move is not to reinstate old-fashioned, class-based 'elocution' classes. These can be divisive and may restrict language rather than free it. What many teachers want is to encourage a move towards ensuring that children of all cultural backgrounds are not disenfranchized because they are not given the language skills that allow them to express their needs clearly and achieve their goals.

There are several organizations that have worked tirelessly over a number of years to promote such work. The English Speaking Board, founded by Christabel Burniston in 1953, has done much to stimulate an interest in spoken language. It offers examinations in oral communication for schools, colleges, commerce and industry. Public speaking festivals and competitions organized by the English Speaking Union have also contributed to the development of the 'oracy' skills of the young people who are fortunate enough to attend a school that participates in these programmes. There are also many local festivals that promote the speaking of verse, prose, broadcasting, and reading as a performance skill. In many schools teachers of English take responsibility for productions and festivals within the school, but with the loss of the specialist the time-consuming task means extra unpaid work for the generous volunteer. (Details of these websites are to be found at the end of the chapter.)

Identifying communication problems in second language speakers

With increasing numbers of children entering schools before having mastered English, the teacher may not be sure whether any difficulties they encounter are present in their first language. It is important to ascertain the fluency of their communication within their first language in order to be able to assess whether a speech delay is simply related to difficulties with a second language or whether it is a more fundamental communication problem also present in the mother tongue. If teachers are concerned about a child's communication skills, then it is important to refer them to Speech and Language Therapy as soon as possible as communication problems can prevent the child from accessing the curriculum.

Spoken English in the curriculum

Oracy Cambridge is a project at Hughes Hall, University of Cambridge, directed by Professor Neil Mercer, which aims to address communication and oracy. On the Oracy Cambridge website, *Oracy@Cambridge*, Mercer states: 'Our research shows that when students learn how to use talk to reason together, they become better at reasoning on their own'. He goes on to advocate spoken language skills being taught in state schools as a way of promoting social equality and life skills such as finding employment ... 'It is also important, in a participatory democracy, that all people – not just those from privileged backgrounds – develop the ability to speak confidently in public, to present effective and persuasive arguments through speech, and to examine critically but constructively the arguments presented by others'.

The website also offers a toolkit which will prove useful to teachers. Undoubtedly the more discursive approach to spoken language allows teacher–student relationships to thrive and become proficient in informal conversational practice, but it is critical to recognize the power of the formal structures that underpin oratory. However, it is not only the learners who need consideration and help with the delivery of language but also the teachers, who in many instances feel that they too would benefit from help both with devising ways of stimulating discussion and verbal analysis. Offering external examinations in Communication and Speech and Drama is one way of extending language skills. Unfortunately, when these are offered they are usually paid for by the families and are not part of the educational offer. Drama teachers sometimes run classes that work towards examinations such as those offered by Trinity College London, LAMDA (London Academy of Music and Dramatic Art) and the English Speaking Board. All three organizations offer examinations in communication skills, and LAMDA and Trinity College London offer examinations in English as a foreign language. Among the organizations they have centres in over 60 countries and offer solo and group examinations. Trinity College, London, for example, has centres in Africa and the Middle East, Asia, the Americas, Australasia and Europe. Some examinations carry a UCAS (Universities and Colleges Admissions Service) tariff and are internationally accepted as credits in many countries, but it is worth checking the status they carry in a specific country before committing to them. Details of webpages for all these examination bodies can be found at the end of this chapter.

Inspiration from arts establishments

Apart from the excellent published material available there are currently many opportunities for teaching staff and students to receive an injection of new ideas and stimuli from outside organizations. Many theatres worldwide receive funding that requires them to offer educational projects or, in some cases, they create an income stream from educational work. It is therefore always worth investigating which arts establishments, such as theatres, museums, art galleries, or orchestras, offer extension work that may nourish the development of oracy.

An example is the London Bubble Theatre Company which offers a project called Speech Bubbles in which school staff, alongside drama practitioners, adopt a child-centered drama approach that encourages communication skills. As many theatres offer schools programmes it is worth contacting your local theatre company to enquire what may be on offer. Some theatre companies run drama workshops on the plays that they produce and offer follow-up packs with suggestions for both written and oral exercises. In the UK, the Royal Shakespeare Company, the Royal National Theatre, Shakespeare's Globe, Young Vic Theatre, Glasgow's Tron Theatre, the National Theatre of Wales, the Birmingham Rep, the Ulster Youth Theatre, and the Konflux Theatre in Northern Ireland, plus many more regional theatres, have proactive Education Departments. The workshops they offer provide a stimulus for discussion rather than a written approach. Some theatres set up residencies in schools as well as offering GCSE, A-Level, and teachers' courses on Shakespeare and contemporary writers. Practical workshops as well as pre- and post-show discussions between creative teams and school groups offer young people insight into the creative process as well as giving them ownership of arts and culture. As for Shakespeare and other classic works, exposure to the fabric of the production and its journey from the text to the stage can remove the fear and formality that often surrounds it. Such interaction between actors, directors, writers and audiences brings together the overlapping worlds of theatre practice, academic scholarship and educational practice. Although the work that they offer may not specifically focus on speech and language, it is practical and drama-based, and will encourage debate in addition to helping the teacher with little experience of drama to explore less conventional approaches to text and language teaching. Theatres in other countries run similar outreach projects which can be found on their websites.

The value of drama as a means of developing self confidence and expressivity is well documented. The opportunity it offers for the development of vocabulary, oracy and debate is equally valuable. Opportunities for young people to become involved in community outreach projects that will require them to use their communication skills are plentiful. Charities in the UK, such as 'Kissing it Better', work with secondary schools and colleges to enhance patient experience in hospitals and care homes. Students are trained and supervized while actively engaging with patients either in conversation or by reading, singing or employing other skills.

Making words enjoyable

Young people are often discouraged when faced with language which to them seems alienating. By entering into language physically, and by speaking words out loud and putting their analytical skills aside for a time, a fuller, more meaningful understanding is achieved. Helpful exercises in this approach can be found in *The Voice Box* (Martin and Darnley, 2013), a box containing exercise cards, and *Your Voice and How to Use it* (Berry, 2000a). Berry's book *The Actor and the Text* (Berry, 2000b) offers exercises for work on literature which can be used to give learners a practical and physical experience of literature. Although the title suggests a book specifically for actors, the exercises can be applied to the classroom. Cicely Berry began working with teachers and young people over 40 years ago and her books are still relevant. Through her need to find ways of making the language of the classics accessible to the young, she has made a seminal contribution to the teaching of language in schools, and formulated an approach that involves the whole class actively entering into the language physically and vocally. The need to cover a syllabus can mean that classes in literature are focused on explaining the narrative and analysing it, rather than gaining understanding by speaking the text aloud.

The experience of speaking the text is all too often neglected in the classroom situation, where the good readers are generally the only ones who get the opportunity, but it is something that can be done in groups and need not intimidate less confident readers. In the drama studio the physical exploration of words is commonplace, but some teachers may find it challenging in the English class.

Beginning a poetry class by physically and vocally exploring the difference between plosive and sustained consonants, or the shapes and resonance of vowels, will soon break down inhibitions and will energize the reading of any poem being discussed. Equally, exploring the number of syllables in a word and discovering which are stressed and which unstressed will expose the rhythms and release the music of the language. Although English and drama classes are the most obvious, a more verbal approach can be explored in most subjects by the introduction of news bulletins, debates, project presentations and interviews in history, music, science, economics, and geography classes.

Finding help for staff

For teachers and lecturers who feel intimidated by having to read verse, prose and dramatic texts aloud, there are classes held through Adult education courses that may be useful, such as a drama group or a public speaking class. Toastmasters and other similar societies offer opportunities to develop skills in formal speaking. Popular at present are groups that offer the opportunity to explore story-telling, oral history and reminiscence, all skills useful to the teacher and skills that can be used to enrich the oral activities within the class. Some people prefer individual classes and in the UK, the Society of Teachers of Speech and Drama provides a list of recognized teachers while similar societies exist in other countries (details of the website can be found at the end of this chapter). There are often workshop advertisements in the theatrical and professional journals available at larger libraries. It is possible that the school's drama teacher, or a teacher with a special interest in drama, may be able to offer support and ideas.

The loss of specialist teachers

A common complaint is that with fewer specialist positions, such as speech and drama teachers and music teachers, many teachers find themselves undertaking a role for which they have had limited preparation, teaching subjects in which they did not originally specialize. Teachers feel justifiably under-confident in teaching a class and a discipline for which they have limited training or qualifications. Some teachers feel a pressure to accept additional duties and are fearful of admitting that they are not able to teach either drama-based work or singing. This is a situation illustrated by the example of a teacher who, because she was the only member of staff in her village school able to play the piano, found herself teaching singing. She commented: 'The worst aspect of teaching singing was that I was so embarrassed at having to demonstrate. Eventually, after becoming extremely anxious about it and on occasions feeling that my throat completely closed up, I went to a wonderful singing teacher at my own expense and gained some confidence. I now enjoy it'. The demands are increasing, and the school should offer the proper training by means of in-service courses for anyone in this position.

In-service training days

When a group of teachers in a school identifies the need for help in a particular area it is usual to approach the school administration and request sponsorship from the staff development fund, or arrange an in-service training or inset day, for which an expert in the field can be brought in. With training for curriculum and procedure issues essential, it can be difficult to find the time and money for what can be seen as basic skills.

Knowledge sharing within schools or school districts is an effective, empowering and cheaper alternative. There are those teachers who have come to the profession because of a natural skill in communication and even in performance. Most secondary schools will have a trained drama teacher who could be asked to run a workshop.

In many institutions, some subjects require skills closer to those of the university lecturer than to those of the classroom teacher, and teaching may involve delivering long tracts of memorized material. In these cases the style of delivery is closer to public speaking, which is explored in Chapters 9 and 12. Developing an interest in debating can enhance this skill, and there are teachers and lecturers who have improved their skills effectively through the experience of having to run a debating society, or by entering groups of students into public speaking competitions. Where only a few teachers from a school require a specific workshop it is sometimes possible to approach the local teachers' centre, or Toastmasters organization, which could provide training.

Special language needs

In the infant school the acquisition of language is rapid and the child explores words and masters syntax through books, stories and play, which become a significant way of making sense of the world. The classroom is an ideal setting for the development of the pupil's ability to use language. It is the place where teachers will recognize early indications of problems in language development or in the acquisition of speech sounds. The child's parents or primary carer, because of either a lack of experience or simply a lack of appreciation of the problem, may have overlooked these signs. Familiarity often makes it difficult to 'isolate' a problem; it is part of the child's repertoire of speech sounds and is, as such, unremarkable. An increasing number of children now attend playgroups and nursery schools where speech and language are fairly closely monitored. Playgroup and nursery school leaders are increasingly aware of the problems that can occur. Fortunately there is ever more awareness of the work of the speech and language therapist/speech pathologist and the intervention that is available, yet there are still a number of children who are overlooked. In the United Kingdom children are taught to read using an approach called synthetic phonics. The phonics approach teaches children to break down words by sounds, rather than recognizing whole words. The UK government's phonics-only approach is not universally admired, some teachers and educationalists advocating a more balanced approach in which other reading strategies are also used.

The problem for the child who is unable to perceive the difference between one sound and another in speech is that it is even more difficult for him or her to perceive the difference between one sound and the other when reading. Children with auditory perpetual difficulties are therefore at a disadvantage when learning to read following this approach, and this may therefore limit their ability to access the curriculum.

Children with limited opportunity for one-to-one conversation, and who demonstrate subtle difficulties with language on either the expressive or receptive side, can be overlooked in a playgroup or nursery setting and their difficulties may only come to light at school entry when there is more need for the child to use language to express more abstract thoughts and ideas. Issues of receptive language difficulty such as semantic relationships, word classes or oral directions, or of expressive language such as recalling sentences, formulating sentences or sentence assembly, can have been overlooked and only become apparent when having to use language in a more precise form.

Although the overarching policy of inclusion in schools is commendable, the increased number of children with special educational needs and disability imposes an increasing burden on teachers and support staff, and may indeed reduce the teacher's ability to find time to focus on children with less severe speech and language disorders.

Although volunteers often provide assistance in the early stages of reading practice, teachers should alert the volunteers to the early warning signals of speech and/or language delay. It is often these 'helpers' and Teaching Assistants who have the most one-to-one contact with the child. The Royal College of Speech and Language Therapists offers advice in recognizing speech and language problems and may be contacted to locate the local clinic or specialist centre.

The Communication Trust has advocated the need for early years staff to be specifically trained in supporting children with delayed speech, language and communication skills, and this requires staff to be able to identify and support children with speech, language, and communication needs (SLCN). Good spoken language skills are strong predictors of later academic success. Children with poor language and literacy development at 5 years are at substantial risk of low achievement at 7 years and beyond (Snowling et al. 2011).

The Communication Trust also states that: 'Many early years staff feel inadequately equipped to help children with language delay with over 60% of teachers reporting they lacked confidence in their ability to meet children's language needs. There is also a wealth of evidence, highlighting the significant and long term impacts on children's literacy, attainment, behaviour, social and emotional development'.

Save The Children UK makes the following observation: 'Without the right support in their early years, children fall behind in their development and start school lacking the crucial skills they need to thrive and learn'. They go on to say: 'In 2015, six children in every reception class in England started school without the early language skills needed to succeed in the classroom.

The effects of falling behind in early development can last a lifetime. The evidence clearly shows that children who start school behind are significantly more likely to remain behind, with consequences that last into adulthood'.

Details of websites for all the above mentioned institutions can be found at the end of this chapter.

Language opportunities in primary and secondary schools

Finding ways of stimulating conversation in the classroom can be challenging. Adolescence, particularly, is a time when alternative views are normal and it is important that schools encourage ideas to be expressed through debate and discussion.

Using texts as a starting point

Speaking the words of others can be the first step to being able to find words for oneself. English literature offers such an enormous variety of wonderfully honed and precisely constructed examples of the expression of every conceivable emotion. When offered to young people for exploration and consideration, verse or prose often releases words and rhythms within individuals and allows their own thoughts to be manifested verbally. The more interactive and vocal the English class becomes the better. Teaching students to appreciate and 'own' literature can be wholly successful only when they experience the speaking of it. Many adolescents have needs that they are not able to express or deal with adequately, such as feelings of rage and grief, huge enthusiasms and devotion to particular groups or individuals. If teachers can help learners and students express their feelings, opinions and needs, and help them to find the words with which to make some sense of their lives, then true education takes place.

Encouraging and, in some cases, reclaiming the art of conversation for young people in the adolescent years can only be beneficial in terms of social interaction, relationships with peers, family and teachers, and with further education, interviews and ultimately with job prospects.

Adolescent frustration which can stem from an inability to express emotions and often leads to violence can, instead of turning in on itself, be channeled through language to become a positive creative force and to lead to a better understanding of self and others. An often quoted line from Thomas Kyd's 16th century play *The Spanish Tragedy* reads 'Where words prevaile [*sic.*] not, violence prevails' and this comment remains current. There are many psychologists, welfare workers and teachers who would agree with this statement, but in the rush to equip young people with writing skills the spoken word often gets neglected. The need to develop the oral skills of society is obvious, but who takes on the burden of the additional teaching?

Although some of the opportunities for the use of verse and prose with adolescents have been mentioned, all age groups from the playgroup upward can adapt and use these approaches. All too often, verse is used only by English and drama teachers but the opportunity to use poetry in history, art, music and social studies, and in fact in almost every class in the school, is often neglected.

Poetry

Poetry offers young people the opportunity to explore their own expressivity, to search for the 'right' word, to consider the order of words, and to play with image and metaphor; it also encourages the personal exploration of deep emotions. Some schools are able to employ a resident poet who works with the learners and students to develop their own poetry skills and to explore different styles and structure. Working with a poet can stimulate and develop the learners' and students' appreciation of language.

Poetry slams

If conventional poetry is considered too 'old fashioned' by some secondary school students, a poetry slam may stimulate interest. Contemporary youth culture embraces spoken word poetry and rap, often with a strong rhythm, that is built around a central pertinent theme. The poetry is often provocative, political, angry and deeply personal, allowing students to explore difficult topics that may be challenging or controversial in adult company or in a more formal setting. For the expressive student with the ability to engage an audience, performance poetry may be a way to nurture a talent for language and inspire an interest in poetic form. Slam poems are devised to be spoken rather than read. They are often constructed in free verse and can be reminiscent of the Beat poets or hip-hop; they can rhyme but essentially there are no rules. Spoken word artists can produce well honed, witty, thought-provoking insight into the youth culture while embracing important universal concerns.

The Poetry Society in the UK currently offers a highly successful and popular project entitled 'SLAMbassadors'. It encourages young people to write a performance poem based on a theme, to video themselves speaking it and then to enter an online competition. Winners get to work with famous spoken word artists.

The Poetry Society has a website dedicated to its youth project and offers a teachers' toolkit. The website states: 'We are seeking life-affirming, angry, soft, political, personal, redemptive, revolutionary and celebratory word art, in an attempt to reclaim lost voices and talent scout the next generation of spoken word artists.'

Contact details for the Poetry Society in the United Kingdom and some international slam poetry organizations can be found at the end of the chapter.

Choral or group speaking

Until the 1970s choral verse was a popular way of teaching children verse in the UK. It lost popularity because it was seen as being taught for all the wrong reasons. It was suspected of being a way of imposing 'Received Pronunciation' (RP) on children who had regional accents and was therefore discarded. There are, however, many positive reasons for encouraging classes to speak together, the most important of all being simply that it offers many children, who are not exposed to verse forms and rhythms, the opportunity to experience the physical joy of speaking poetry. Other benefits include exposure to alternative language structures, metaphor, onomatopoeia, vocabulary, and imagery. There is always a danger that the teacher will feel the need to make the children sound 'correct' rather than allowing them to feel the energy and the sound-scape of the language, the sheer enjoyment of telling the story, and communicating it to the audience. The act of speaking together develops empathy between members of the group and a sense of team spirit similar to that developed through participation in sport. The demands made by the exercise go far beyond the simple act of memorizing words.

The speaking of well selected verse demands a feeling for rhythm that informs the learner's own speech and writing, and their appreciation of rhythm in verse and prose. It offers a valuable experience of performance for the shy child. The practical approach of speaking language rather than analysing it provides an organic and physical engagement with language.

A group can also explore verse by taking a line each around the classroom, responding to the vocal energy of the words and of each other, and developing a 'communal voice'. Working towards sharing of work with other classes and parents can be an enriching experience for all, but it is sometimes a mistake to concentrate on the performance of group verse rather than simply speaking it for enjoyment. The process should always be more important than the product. When choosing verse to speak chorally, look for dynamic language with strong rhythms and sound patterns.

Speaking words together that have been carefully chosen to be part of a well shaped and honed structure takes language beyond the page and 'into the mouth', so that the learners and students experience it viscerally. The speaking of powerful words can promote awareness that words have enormous power and influence to change people, situations and ultimately, lives.

Singing

Most singing teachers do a wonderful job in the musical life of the school. Stories still exist, however, of children who have been adversely affected, and in some cases scarred, by thoughtless and often ignorant remarks. Some teachers recalled humiliating remarks made to them by class or singing teachers about their supposed 'inability' to sing. These remarks were followed by suggestions that they should not sing but rather, 'mouth' the words. Such suggestions are never child-centred but are usually concerned with the teacher's, or the head teacher's, desire to produce a 'polished' performance for an adult audience. Telling a child who finds maths difficult simply to refrain from completing the lesson would be seen as irresponsible, so why should it be acceptable to prevent some children from singing when what they need to improve their pitching is more practice, not less. With enough practice and positive guidance and encouragement, the child who pitches normally in speech can be given the confidence to pitch accurately in song. Singing should be a natural, joyous and fundamental part of every child's education and, as with choral verse, the process should be more important than the product.

A study at the Institute of Education (Ward, 2003) showed that parents who criticize or laugh at their children's attempts to sing or play an instrument risk turning the children off music for life. The study, mirroring the teacher's anecdotal comments above, suggested that an adult's dislike of music can usually be traced back to a 'disapproving experience' of making music as a child, either at home or at school. The researchers at the Institute of Education said that even a throwaway remark from a parent or teacher can 'foster a sense of childhood or adolescent musical inadequacy and shame that can persist into old age'. (Details of the website containing the article can be found at the end of the chapter.)

The teaching of singing to young children, who in many cases have hearing that is not yet sufficiently sophisticated to pitch accurately, should also involve teaching them to listen through a series of auditory training exercises. These lessons in listening will have a positive effect in many other areas of school life. Singing can also provide excellent practice in speech sounds because definition is required and produced when the children are committed to the act of singing.

The singing lesson, as with the choral speaking lesson, offers a wonderful opportunity to establish the essence of easy, free, spontaneous voice use.

Children can be encouraged to align their posture and stand with the weight on both feet and with a long spine. They can be taught to 'breathe down' rather than to 'take a big breath', to release the shoulders, relax the jaw and keep the head balanced and aligned on the top of the spine. The opportunity to establish these fundamental postural principles should not be lost. Being part of a group that is involved in the creation of communal sound is a wonderful experience whatever the age of the learner or student. Much has been written about the act of singing and any reduction of this essentially primal social and cultural activity is to be deeply regretted. In selecting material for song, as for verse, it is important to reflect not only the majority school population but also to embrace minority cultures within the school. Music and verse can greatly enhance empathy with other cultures and understanding of other countries. The singing of traditional songs allows children to enter into other musical and narrative traditions and to develop an interest in story-telling that may be lacking in the modern family unit. It can provide a useful way of extending work on other languages and may naturally engage with different subject areas, such as history and geography.

The value of singing goes beyond building vocabulary, memory training and technical aspects of breath, pitch, communication and precision of sounds because, as with all language, its delivery is a gestalt, involving body, breath, mind, intention, rhythm, musicality, and interpretation. It develops not only musicality but also the interpersonal and ensemble skills of group timing, anticipation and co-operation. For many children the act of group speaking or singing allows them a great deal of freedom to explore their own creative powers and imagination. It is inclusive and brings a sense of companionship, and it provides the opportunity to be in a team and to perform safely without exposure.

Suggestions for language based activities for the classroom

Keep 'showing and telling'

Everyone has memories of the 'Show and Tell' exercise in primary school. It has great value as it develops basic communication skills and encourages children to begin to present their thoughts and ideas to an audience. The demands the exercise makes will be those faced in everyday adult working life. The verbal skills gained will be as useful in adult life as skills in mathematics, science, and written English. These skills include:

- engaging an audience;
- physically taking command of the space;
- critical thinking;
- creating a narrative or a sequential structure;
- putting across an opinion by developing an argument and debating the pros and cons;
- answering questions;
- using the voice artistically and applying the elements of emphasis, pause, and other aspects of modulation;
- becoming familiar with the social etiquette involved in exchanging ideas such as not interrupting and turn taking;
- listening attentively to others speaking and formulating and asking questions.

Developing this into an exercise for older students is easy. Simply modify the exercise by asking them to:

- demonstrate how a technical object works or is constructed;
- invent a unique or imaginary way of using a simple object;
- trace the history of an object;
- bring an object that has had a significant impact on society such as a postage stamp, a fork, a wheel, etc.; or

- describe the personal significance an object has for you, such as a letter, a gift, a photograph, or a toy.

There are numerous ways of stimulating communication in an enjoyable but challenging way. While the language or drama class provides a perfect environment for verbal and physical communication, all subjects can become a focus and starting point for verbal and vocal extension.

Classroom communication games

Five facts

Ask the group to divide into pairs. One student is the speaker, the other is the listener. The speaker tells the listener five facts about themselves in one minute. The pair swaps roles and repeats the exercise. They then introduce each other to the group using the information they have gleaned.

What is it?

Divide the group into pairs. Give each student a picture of an object such as an animal, a kitchen utensil, a landscape, a machine, a building, a bridge, a ship, a busy harbour, a crime scene, etc. Ask students to describe the scene, without saying what it is or showing their partner, and offer as much information as possible about what they see. Give the activity a time limit. Suggest they verbally create the atmosphere and emotional energy of the picture. The partner/listener has to guess the object. The listener can ask questions.

The game can be extended to require the listener to repeat as many of the details of the photograph as they can remember to the group.

How to...

Ask the group to prepare detailed verbal instructions on how to:

- bake a cake;
- roast a chicken;
- cook their favourite meal;
- make their own festive/birthday card;
- create a vegetable garden;

- change a car or bicycle tyre;
- apply for a passport; or
- open a bank account.

NB: Give a time limit and strongly enforce it.

Vocabulary game

Create word cards. Each card should have an unusual word printed on it.

Ask everyone to look up the meaning of their word and use it in a sentence. With older students, ask them to research the etymology of the word. Extend the game by asking the group to swap words and produce new sentences.

The game can be further extended by asking the group to improvise a group story and to include as many of the group's words as they can. Once a new word has been included, another student continues to improvise the story. The story can be told to the rest of the class.

A baton can be passed around the group to indicate it is another person's turn or a gentle touch on the shoulder can be used.

The extension game

In pairs, ask the group to begin with one partner making a statement such as 'I bought an apple'. The next partner adds to this by saying 'I bought a red apple'.

As the statement moves between the partners it grows, e.g., 'I bought a beautiful red apple', and so on, adding words like delicious, scrumptious, worm-ridden, etc.

Group story telling

Select a well known story such as Cinderella or a clichéd phrase such as 'It was a dark and stormy night' and sitting in groups of up to 10 go round the group with each individual adding their own sentence. In the case of a well known story they do not need to repeat the original plot line but can fabricate their own ideas.

Group and solo improvisation

Improvisation is a useful skill to develop in the classroom as being unscripted it develops the ability to 'think on one's feet,' work as a team, problem solve, and encourage creativity. It also builds vocabulary and demands that language is accessed spontaneously. Subjects should be age appropriate and can allow young people to safely experience difficult situations they encounter in their everyday lives, or will do as young adults. The skills and confidence gained will be helpful in interviews and other impromptu situations in life. Above all, improvisation, once mastered, is great fun and allows the imagination and inventiveness full rein.

There are a number of excellent books on the art of improvisation which can be found in the further reading section at the end of the chapter. Most books on classroom drama contain improvisation guidelines and suggestions for suitable subjects and situations.

Poem share

Ask the learners or students to choose a poem and to tell the group why they enjoyed it. They should read at least a verse of the poem to the class.

Class poetry slam

Ask the class to create their own piece of performance poetry to share with the rest of the group. This can be done individually or as a small group. Provide some time for writing and rehearsal. Examples of performance poetry can be found online and used to illustrate the form, inspire form and inspire young poets.

Book reviews

Spoken book, television, theatre, or film reviews can become the focus for an exercise in communication. This can be undertaken by an individual or a small group, so that the structure and content of the review can be discussed and different aspects and opinions can be presented by members of the group.

I enjoy/dislike

Ask every member of the group to make a statement about something they either enjoy or dislike, and to justify the statement with *because* . . . Initially, only one sentence should be spoken. Thereafter the sentence limit can be extended and the argument expanded to allow for greater expression of ideas and freer use of language.

What is your opinion on . . .

Give the group an age-appropriate subject.

This could range from simple ideas, such as school uniforms and pocket money, to more challenging subjects, such as immigration, university degrees, apprenticeships, nature conservation, women's rights, human rights, or other current social and political issues.

Ask the class to make notes on their opinion of the subject. Allow a specified time such as a minute to make notes. Create a rules and boundaries structure to avoid interruption, insult or disruption and to encourage listening, questioning, sensitivity to the feelings and ideas of others, and polite and considerate social interaction.

Your turn to be teacher

Offer regular opportunities for members of the group to research a subject and then teach it. This can be done as a short solo exercise or better still, in groups, where a number of students take on different aspects or sections of the subject.

Current affairs

Focusing on current affairs creates an opportunity for expression; it also increases general knowledge, political and civic awareness, and prepares young people for participation in the democratic process. A class can be divided into groups and each group given a subject to research. The research could be limited to a single library lesson or extended over a number of weeks to include interviews, recordings, photographs and diagrams. Topics can be drawn from national or local newspapers. Once researched, the group can return to the class and give a group presentation. Topics are endless but could include:

- An interview with:
  - town planners to find out how local planning decisions are made,
  - members of the parks and recreation department,
  - the local Member of Parliament (or similar government official depending on the system in your country), or
  - local residents affected by planning decisions including new roads, housing developments, supermarkets.
- A visit to:
  - the local council to find out its responsibilities and how it operates,
  - a local radio station,
  - the local newspaper,
  - an animal sanctuary,
  - a local place of historic interest,
  - a local place of worship (other than your own) and finding out about the religion and traditions of the faith.
- Meeting with:
  - members of the local fire department,
  - local charities to discover how they use their donations,
  - immigrants and learning about their lives before and after they left their home country.
- Finding out:
  - about the life and careers of priests, farmers, lawyers, members of the police force, scientists, traffic wardens, professional athletes, actors, quantity surveyors, or architects,
  - how recycling is done in your area.

Advertisements

After observing advertisements in magazines and on television and listening to the radio, analyse the commonly used structures such as repetition, antithesis, alliteration, and the three point list; ask learners or students to write their own advertisements and perform them in groups.

Speechmaking

Speechmaking can start in the primary school and develop with more formal structures in secondary school. Suggest that the learners or students compose and deliver an age-appropriate speech on a subject. The choice of subjects is endless but these are some suggested titles:

- Primary/elementary schools:
  - Why I like baking, gardening, reading, etc.
  - My holiday or my dream holiday.
  - The responsibilities of owning a pet.
  - Moving house.
  - What I would like to do when I leave school.
  - My hobby.
  - My elderly friend.
  - Why we need to recycle.
  - My hero/heroine.
  - My little sister, brother, or cousin.

- Secondary/high schools:
  - Accepting a prize.
  - Saying farewell to a co-worker or fellow student.
  - Congratulating someone on winning an award.
  - Toasting the wedding party.
  - Offering an apology.
  - Supporting the election of someone to the local council.
  - Explaining the value of regular exercise.
  - Offering a perspective on social media and its impact.
  - Campaigning for election to the student union or other board/council.
  - Nominating someone for a position of responsibility.

- Campaigning or fundraising for a cause, for example: wildlife conservation, local dog home, community hospital, hospice, an aspect of medical research, local amateur theatre, etc.
- Seeking financial backing for a business initiative.

Inventions

Ask the group to speak about an invention they would like to see and say why it would be a good idea. Illustrations can be used. The speech should be approximately 1 minute long for the young and less confident, but could be adjusted accordingly. Time limits should be strongly adhered to as they require more disciplined thinking and succinct language.

Famous speeches

A wonderful way to explore and understand rhetoric and good communication is to present famous political speeches. Excellent examples of these can be found online. For example, a history class could present some of the speeches from the period they are studying, including both inspiring and controversial speeches.

Ask the class members to select a speech (or extract) and perform it for the class. The student or another member of the class could introduce the speech, giving it an historical, social and political context. Allow discussion of the content and delivery afterwards.

Encourage students to explore international speeches as well as those delivered by speakers from their own heritage. They need not necessarily agree with the politics and should be encouraged to express their own opinions afterwards.

Although the majority of historical speeches are by men there are wonderful, lesser known speeches by women. Contemporary speeches by women are readily available. Suggested subjects include:

- human rights;
- women's suffrage;
- abolition of slavery;

- contemporary politics;
- scientific research;
- early exploration;
- space exploration;
- speeches from the world wars and other conflicts.

The subjects are numerous and can be chosen to reflect the culture and abilities of the group.

Word games

Ask the school to invest in popular word games such as *Articulate*™. It is a team game that provides a wonderful opportunity to communicate verbally. One member has to describe the word printed on a card to their team without mentioning it. The others in the team have to guess the word. The aim is for the team to guess as many words as possible in 30 seconds. The describer cannot mention the word but can say 'rhymes with' or 'sounds like'. If the word is 'bridge' it could be described as 'a structure that enables people to get from one side of a river to the other side' or it could be said that 'one of these can be found in Sydney Harbour'. It is ideal for a rainy day when the group must remain indoors during break. Games such as Charades encourage physical expression by the person performing the actions and encourage the 'guessers' to search for words and match words to actions. It is also a great 'ice breaker'.

Debating

Debating is a valuable way of developing language and advocacy skills, argument, confidence, listening, and eloquence. It also teaches discipline, organization, and respect for others. There is good advice online on how to stage a classroom debate or start an extracurricular debating society.

For those who wish to debate at competition level there are inter-school and international competitions in which to participate. In the UK, the Institute of Ideas runs an annual Debating Matters Competition and offers resources and guidance for schools new to debating. Other helpful organizations promoting debating and holding competitions are The Cambridge Union Schools

Debating Competition, The English Speaking Union Schools' Mace, and Debate Mate. Debate Mate provides workshops for teachers and students led by university student mentors, all of whom are experienced debaters. Similar organizations exist in most countries.

The details of the websites of all these organizations can be found at the end of this chapter.

School radio or television news

Developing media skills can be educational on many levels from technical production to presentation. While some schools have facilities that can be adapted for school radio or filming, a studio is not essential. It is possible to record on mobile/cell phones, or simply stage an unrecorded presentation for the class.

Ask some members of the group to be presenters and others to be reporters. They can report on anything that is age appropriate. Presentations can be researched as a project over a number of days, or improvised if the group is experienced and confident with improvisation. The choice of subjects is limitless and can include:

- weather;
- international news;
- cultural events;
- local news;
- politics;
- arts; or
- sport.

If the school or college can support its own radio station for a short period each day, magazine programmes can focus on community and school events and sports results, and can contain interviews and competitions. Budding disc jockeys can provide music. Once up and running, skills will be passed from one student to another, but initially some training will be needed in the use of equipment, presentation, programming, and organization. It may be possible to contact a local radio station or hospital radio for advice. These projects should be enjoyable and foster a desire to communicate.

BBC School Report

A popular innovation has been the BBC project 'School Report' which celebrated its 10th annual News Day in March 2016. The project encourages school children to research and present topical news items and in so doing, learn to 'find, gather, write and broadcast' news for radio and television. Information, ideas and resources are given to teachers. Even if participating in this worthwhile project is not possible, simplified versions of the exercises can be adapted and developed in most schools.

The BBC project 'School Report' shows what can be achieved and how enthusiastic and inspired participants can be. The website details can be found at the end of this chapter.

Competitions and festivals

Encourage talented students to enter public speaking competitions, eisteddfodau or local arts festivals. These festivals offer students the opportunity to practice their skills in public speaking, sight reading, poetry and drama. Groups can be entered for choral verse, so that even the less confident members of a group can enjoy the experience.

If you are unsure of where UK festivals take place, the Federation of Festivals has a webpage, details of which can be found at the end of the chapter. Similar websites exist in other countries and can be searched for by using phrases such as 'arts festivals', 'speech and drama festivals', 'music and drama festivals', or 'eisteddfodau'.

Chapter outline

- Vocal persona
- The effects of technology
- Spoken English in the curriculum
- Ideas from the arts
- Making words physical
- Finding help
- In service training days
- Special language needs
- Language opportunities in the primary or secondary school
- Poetry
- Poetry slam
- Choral or group speaking
- The loss of specialist teachers
- Singing
- Suggestions for language based activities for the classroom

References and further reading

BBC School Report. Available at: <http://www.bbc.co.uk/schoolreport/teacher_resources [Accessed August 2017].

Berry C. 2000a. *Your Voice and How to Use it*. London: Virgin Books.

Berry C. 2000b. *The Actor and the Text*. London: Virgin Books.

Bivens-Tatum W. 2008. The evolution of a teaching persona. *Academic Librarian* December 2008. Available at: <https://blogs.princeton.edu/librarian/2008/12/the_evolution_of_a_teaching_persona/> [Accessed August 2017].

The Cambridge Union, Schools' Debating Competition. Available at: <http://cambridg-eschools.cus.org/> [Accessed August 2017].

The Communication Trust. Available at: <https://www.thecommunicationtrust.org.uk/media/39152/consultation_on_early_education_and_childcare_staff_deployment.pdf> [Accessed August 2017].

Debate Mate. Available at: <https://debatemate.com/home/> [Accessed August 2017].

Debating Matters. Available at: <http://www.debatingmatters.com/> [Accessed August 2017].

English Speaking Board. Available at: <http://esbuk.org/> [Accessed August 2017].

English Speaking Union. Available at: <http://www.esu.org/> [Accessed August 2017].

The English Speaking Union, Schools' Mace. Available at: <http://www.esu.org/our-work/schools-mace> [Accessed August 2017].

Federation of Festivals. Available at: <www.federationoffestivals.org.uk/festivals-a-z> [Accessed August 2017].

Kissing it Better Charity. Available at: <http://www.kissingitbetter.co.uk/> [Accessed August 2017].

KQED, Mind Shift. Available at: <https://ww2.kqed.org/mindshift/2016/10/03/why-the-art-of-speaking-should-be-taught-alongside-math-and-literacy/> [Accessed August 2017].

Kyd T. 2010. *The Spanish Tragedy*. Calvo C and Tronch J (eds). London: Arden Early Modern Drama.

LAMDA. Available at: <www.lamda.org.uk> [Accessed August 2017].

McKnight KS and Scruggs M. 2008. *The Second City Guide to Improv in the Classroom: using improvisation to teach skills and boost learning*. San Francisco, CA: Jossey-Bass.

Martin S and Darnley L. 2012. *The Voice Box*. London: Speechmark.

Oracy@Cambridge. Available at: <www.hughes.cam.ac.uk> [Accessed August 2017].

Palmer S. 2007. *Toxic Childhood: How the modern world is damaging our children and what we can do about it*. London: Orion.

Poetry Society UK. Available at: <http://poetrysociety.org.uk/> [Accessed August 2017].

The Royal College of Speech and Language Therapists. Available at: <https://www.rcslt.org/> [Accessed August 2017].

Save the Children. Available at: <http://blogs.savethechildren.org.uk/2016/05/why-government-must-recognise-that-children-start-learning-before-school/> [Accessed August 2017].

Shepherd, A. *Times Educational Supplement*. Available at: <https://www.tes.com/article.aspx?storycode=21135848> [Accessed August 2017].

Society of Teachers of Speech and Drama. Available at: <http://www.stsd.org.uk/> [Accessed August 2017].

Snowling MJ, Hulme C, Bailey, *et al.* (2011) Language and literacy attainment of pupils during early years and through KS2: Does teacher assessment at five provide a valid measure of children's current and future educational attainments? *Research Report DFE-RR172a.* Department for Education. Available at: <http://www.education.gov.uk/publications/eOrderingDownload/DFE-RR172a.pdf> [Accessed August 2017].

Speech Bubbles. Available at: <http://www.londonbubble.org.uk/projectpage/speech-bubbles/> [Accessed August 2017].

Spolin V. 1986. *Theater Games for the Classroom: A teacher's handbook.* Evanston, IL: Northwestern University Press.

Sure Start. Available at: <https://www.gov.uk/find-sure-start-childrens-centre> [Accessed August 2017].

Toastmasters. Available at: <https://www.toastmasters.org> [Accessed August 2017].

Trinity College London. Available at: <www.trinitycollege.com/drama> [Accessed August 2017].

Ward L. 2003. Mocking can scar children. *The Guardian*, 28 October 2003. Available at: <https://www.theguardian.com/uk/2003/oct/28/childprotection.children> [Accessed August 2017].

Wilson K. 2008. *Drama and Improvisation.* Oxford: Oxford University Press.

International Poetry Slam societies: Suggested links

Australia. Available at: <http://www.australianpoetryslam.com/about/> [Accessed August 2017].

Europe. Available at: <http://beslam.be/euroslam/> [Accessed August 2017].

Hong Kong. Available at: <https://www.facebook.com/PoetryOutLoudHK/> [Accessed August 2017].

India. Available at: <https://www.facebook.com/events/1710748639174952/> [Accessed August 2017].

Singapore. Available at: <http://www.wordforward.org/singapore-poetry-slamtrade.html> [Accessed August 2017].

South Africa. Available at: <http://www.goethe.de/ins/za/prj/spw/plc/job/enindex.htm> [Accessed August 2017].

United Kingdom: The Poetry Society, Slambassadors. Available at: <https://slam.poetrysociety.org.uk/about/> [Accessed August 2017].

United States of America Available at: <http://poetryslam.com/> [Accessed August 2017].

9

Beyond the teaching role

This chapter explores some of the additional duties and demands that educators may have to take on as part of their professional role. Educators working with all age groups deal with the need to change their communication style frequently, adapting to the needs of the moment. Situations can change quickly and it can become necessary to respond by adapting the style of delivery. At other times the new role is anticipated and can be planned for.

The chapter offers practical guidance and is intended to provide pragmatic user-friendly solutions and suggestions, some of which come into the 'quick-fix' category while others will require longer-term attention to achieve lasting change.

The teacher as orator

Within this role the teacher may be expected to address the school assembly, lead the prayers, give a moral speech, convey daily information to the assembled school, address a governors' meeting, welcome the audience to a play or music evening and possibly, address a gathering of parents on matters pertaining to the children's education, such as changes in education policy, secondary and further education options, and fundraising.

In order to give a good speech it is most important to take time for preparation. Hoping that when the time comes it will be possible to 'come up with something' will not work. The fear of having to speak is halved the moment preparation begins. With confidence the voice will remain controlled, although obviously a little tension or 'stage fright' is natural and even useful because it provides an adrenaline rush and gives the 'edge' that may be described as 'sharpening the wits'. Teachers and lecturers address groups all day, every day; it is what they are good at. Nevertheless, this can sometimes be forgotten in the anxiety of the more formal arena of 'giving a speech'.

The use of a clearly defined note structure along the lines of a composition structure, with a beginning, middle and end, is advisable. As a useful 'rough' measure, the middle of the talk should carry 60% of the message, and the beginning and end 20% each. It is a great help to both speaker and listener if the main points can be clearly signaled and a framework developed that contains the focus of the speech. Obviously the skills of oratory are specialized and much has been written that will help those who wish to extend their competence in this area. At the most simplistic level the recommendation to use the Aristotelian triptych 'tell them what you're going to tell them, tell them, then tell them what you've told them' is valuable. In other words: introduce the subject, develop the subject and then summarize it for the audience. It is also important to 'get the audience on side' from the beginning and to establish a relationship and common ground, no matter how difficult the subject matter. As mentioned in **Chapter 8**, oratory is complex and cannot be condensed into a few paragraphs. For those who wish to become accomplished public speakers there are excellent books on the subject, and some titles can be found at the end of this chapter under further reading.

Introducing and thanking speakers

Often, the teacher's duty is to welcome a speaker or to thank one. It is always advisable to undertake some research beforehand. The speaker's background, achievements and connection with the educational institution should be included in the introduction. If the teacher's duty is to thank them, notes should be made during the speech and the salient and most memorable points mentioned at the end. Even an informal occasion such as an address by a guest speaker can produce considerable tension in the individual who has to officiate. The voice can feel as if it has 'seized up' in these moments of pressure, or it may be difficult to focus on what the speaker is saying when anticipating having to thank them. The question is, what can be done in terms of self-help? The answer is, quite a lot.

The most important point is that the speech should have been practiced a number of times, preferably to a real 'audience', be it a partner, a friend or a colleague if possible. It is important for any speech to be spoken aloud, not for it to be practiced silently or gone over in the individual's head. If there is no opportunity to practice with an audience, a mobile/cell phone or digital recorder may be used for playback purposes, but without an audience it will be difficult for the individual to rehearse the experience of communicating with people rather than listening to him/herself speak.

When rehearsing, make sure that the body is well aligned with the weight distributed across both feet. Shifting the weight from one foot to another gives the audience the immediate impression that the speaker is ill at ease. Standing firmly but without tension and comfortably 'occupying the space' not only looks better but also, allows a sense of being in control.

As a general rule it is not advisable for speakers to carry a lot of papers to the podium with them. There is a danger that notes may be lost among other papers or, worse still, that they may be dropped. Most importantly, a speech should not be learnt 'parrot fashion'; it is important to have notes as guidance so that if, through anxiety, part of the 'script' is forgotten, the speaker can glance at the notes as a prompt to move to the next point. When speaking it is important to speak directly to the audience not at them; wide ranging eye contact should be made with members of the audience, but do not fix on a specific individual. Time should be allowed for pauses so that significant points can be digested. Above all, the voice should maintain the speaker's natural inflection and intonation pattern. It is important to remember that the odd slip is not the end of the world; the audience is generally on the side of the speaker and wants them to succeed.

If you find that you are expected to make speeches on a regular basis and are intimidated by the idea, or conversely if you really enjoy the role, you could join a branch of Toastmasters in order to further your skills. Information can be found on their website under 'Find a Club Near You'. The link to the websites can be found at the end of the chapter.

The following suggestions may be useful when preparing a speech:

- Allow enough time for adequate preparation.
- Acknowledge your audience.
- A smile will relax you and engage your audience.
- Relax shoulders and release tension in the jaw, knees, arms, and feet.
- Stand well with weight evenly distributed.
- Use simple notes that will guide you through your speech.
- Research the background and achievements of the individual or individuals you will be introducing.
- If you are thanking a speaker, listen carefully to the speech and make notes on the content so that you can refer to specific points.
- If you are using a microphone, ask for a sound check before the event begins.

If there is a microphone available, it is important to ensure that it has been tested and that it works, before it is used. Audiences find it disconcerting when a speaker taps a microphone and asks whether they can be heard, and the process will often undermine the speaker's confidence. A trial run is very important, allowing the speaker to find the best position in relation to the microphone and experimenting to achieve the most acceptable volume. Being too close will causing 'popping' and being too far away will dissipate the sound and disengage the audience. Nothing is worse for an audience than to be blasted with sound, or for the speaker to find that most of the speech has been inaudible. Further suggestions for the correct use of a microphone are offered later in the chapter, and additional suggestions and practice material for speeches can be found in **Chapter 12.**

The teacher as sports coach

Within this role the teacher may be expected to work out of doors in all weathers, shout to encourage the team, issue instructions, and caution unruly behaviour. It might also include teaching swimming in a large indoor pool with a very poor acoustic, being a cricket umpire during the hayfever season, teaching physical education, gym or dance, and having to speak while demonstrating.

A problem produced by the need to vocalize while exercising is that less breath support can be given to the voice when lying down than when standing up; however, much of the yoga, Pilates, and gym teachers' work is demonstration led and floor work predominates. The number of exercise teachers who experience voice problems is high and far outweighs that of dance teachers. When music accompanies exercise classes the volume should be turned down or the teacher should use a microphone.

Sports duties are likely to present the most vocal challenges. The cold of a sports field or stadium is a problem because, as has already been noted, when people are cold they tend to raise their shoulders and tighten the neck and jaw, pull back the head and fold the arms across their body. This physical position is not conducive to easy efficient voice production. The open space is another problem. There are no hard vibrating surfaces for sound to bounce off, so the voice fades as it travels over the distance and as a result, the teacher shouts. Shouting in itself is not a problem; it is after all a natural activity and children shout joyously in the playground. Unfortunately, the 'art of shouting' is something many adults in the Western world have lost. In many cultures shouting is still commonplace and it is not seen as aggressive, but in British and some other cultures, it is perceived as being related to anger or frustration. Chapter 10 looks at producing volume in a healthy manner, a technique well worth learning for anyone who needs to project loudly over distance, over noise, or out of doors.

Some helpful suggestions when using the voice on the field are:

- If possible use a megaphone. This may be quickly made with a piece of cardboard. If this is not possible, the hand should be cupped around the mouth and the speaker should try to 'call' rather than shout.

- Remember that this is not a war, it is a sport. Keeping a healthy voice is much more likely if a sense of humour is retained. In laughter the voice is wonderfully free; the joyous 'Yes!' produced by a supporter when the team suddenly makes a brilliant move after playing abysmally is very different from the exasperated 'Come on!' before the successful event.
- Set out clear boundaries about behavior and enforce them. This will avoid the need to shout while attempting to maintain order.
- Make sure students keep in sight and ask them to respond to visual commands such as hand or flag signals.
- Wear warm clothing, scarves and gloves to keep warm; warm up if necessary by exercising. Take a team near to a wall or keep them close in order to use a more conversational voice level when coaching.
- Do not battle against the wind; if the wind is blowing it is unlikely that the speaker will be easily audible. Children are more likely to understand a speaker who is clearly mouthing the words. The use of a control, such as a whistle, or flags, or a signalling system that is understood by the children, is recommended in order to preserve vocal health in difficult sporting situations.

The teacher who has to teach swimming has the least enviable job! The acoustics in indoor pools are invariably poor because of the abundance of hard surfaces and high ceilings. Often they are echo chambers and the space becomes incredibly noisy, particularly if the classes take place while public or shared sessions are occurring simultaneously. In such a situation it is difficult to offer helpful advice because many teachers report not only that it is a most difficult task but also that it causes considerable vocal tiredness. Some teachers have reported that with improved voice production techniques and the use of non-verbal ways of controlling the group, it has been possible to cope better. As with field sports, the use of a control to minimize voice use is important; whistles can be high-pitched enough to pierce the noisy acoustic, although problems occur if other teachers use them in shared sessions. Using a flag to get children to swim to the side can be effective, but often a sound signal will be needed as well. A variety of signals should be taught to the children, e.g., one long blast means 'stop', two short blasts means 'come to the side'.

Small children and non-swimmers should be taught only in a quiet environment and in small groups. All children should be clearly instructed on what to do when they have completed a length so that they look to the teacher for advice before proceeding. It is pointless to expect children to hear anything when their heads are in the water.

Teachers should watch their posture as they lean towards swimmers, bending from the knees rather than leaning from the waist. It is advisable to wear suitable comfortable clothing and shoes.

It is important to remember that even children, who seldom lose their voices, can be hoarse after a gala. This is because the noise rebounds off the hard surfaces and supporters find themselves shouting louder and louder in order to hear themselves. All that those in the water hear is a roar of sound. It is in this highly competitive atmosphere that problems can occur. The usual advice about drinking water applies here too because pools are usually overheated. If possible, teachers who are not involved in the gala should be encouraged to keep discipline on the bus going back to school in order to prevent additional vocal damage.

In these testing vocal situations:

- Apply your knowledge of posture, breath, and voice production to your teaching.
- Be aware of head–neck alignment, particularly when cold or when cheering on your team.
- Be prepared for all weathers. Keep a scarf, warm jacket, and comfortable shoes at school or college.
- If you suffer from allergies keep an antihistamine spray or tablets on hand.
- Carry drinking water.
- Avoid 'competing' with extraneous noise.

- Use a megaphone or other 'control' such as a flag or whistle.
- Encourage visual forms of communication.
- Set clear boundaries about discipline in swimming pools, gym halls, or sports fields.
- Monitor posture.
- Maintain relaxed posture while using volume.
- Avoid shouting and where possible, gather groups around you in a sheltered position.
- Develop your ability to use high volume and 'shout safely'. Further exercises for this can be found in **Chapter 10**.

All the above suggestions also apply to indoor spaces with high ceilings and hard surfaces, such as squash and badminton courts.

The teacher as entertainer

Within this role the teacher may be expected to perform as the disc jockey at a noisy disco, call the dances at a fundraising barn dance, make the public address announcements at fetes, and perform, often unwillingly, at leavers' parties! Of all these activities the most vocally dangerous is to shout above the noise of the disco; a microphone should always be used in such instances. Always check the microphone levels before the event and ask someone to feed back if levels are too loud or quiet. Teachers who are not happy in this role should try to avoid being forced into entertaining by offering to contribute in another way. Many extroverts really enjoy and embrace their role as entertainer; for many others it is their worst fear. There may be members of the school board or parent teachers' association who will welcome the opportunity.

Some helpful suggestions for 'entertainers' are:

- Check posture if you are playing instruments and singing at the same time.
- Make sure you are given rehearsal time in the venue.
- Ask for help with setting up and clearing away.

- Do not be forced into entertaining if you do not enjoy it and find it intimidating and stressful.
- Use a microphone if possible.

The following section offers information on the use of a microphone.

Microphone technique

In certain instances the use of a microphone can be very helpful. More teachers are using microphones than ever before. In some cultures they are the norm rather than the exception. In the UK they are more likely to be found in universities than classrooms unless a student is using a hearing aid or there is a sound field system in the classroom.

Microphones are not the answer to all vocal issues and voice care, and where possible training should be given on the proper technique for their use, otherwise they could simply exacerbate the problem. The teacher could easily become reliant on the microphone rather than improving their vocal technique. It is essential that the vocal support and clarity of articulation is equally good, with or without a microphone.

The quality of the equipment is also important. Good quality equipment should be sourced and it can be expensive. It is important that not only a good microphone is used but also, that the amplification system is of good quality and properly set up. We have all been at school fetes, in supermarkets, and sat in railway stations or airports where announcements have been completely inaudible and incomprehensible, simply adding to the noise level.

Using a microphone requires a sound test in order to balance the level to suit the space. The microphone needs to be held at an appropriate distance from the mouth and speech needs to be supported by the breath and clearly articulated. If you 'mumble' into a microphone all you will achieve is louder mumbling.

Consider the following when using a microphone:

- If a technician is available, involve him in the setting up of the microphone and ask how the system operates.

- If possible ask a technician or a member of staff to listen to you and offer feedback on the vocal quality. If sound is too loud, or if windows are open, noise could carry to another classroom.
- When using a fixed microphone at a lectern it is important to position yourself in front of the microphone and with the microphone pointed in the direction of the mouth, rather than at the ceiling or chest.
- It might be necessary to adjust the microphone before you begin speaking. This is especially important if you are following a speaker of a different height.
- When adjusting the microphone avoid touching the woven steel casing or removable windscreen as this would create noisy feedback.
- Whenever possible, make adjustments before you start rather than having to interrupt your presentation, performance, or speech once you have started.
- Avoid 'poking' the head forward in an effort to direct the voice into the microphone. This will affect your vocal quality and detract from your ability to engage your audience. You can maintain an open posture up to approximately 18–25 cm (approximately 7–10 inches) from the microphone. While being aware of the need to direct speech into the microphone, relax the shoulders and avoid a tense, fixed body position.
- When using a portable hand-held microphone, avoid holding the microphone too near the mouth as this will distort the sound and create unpleasant feedback and 'popping' on plosive consonants.
- Whether using a hand-held or fixed microphone, remember you are communicating with an audience and look at them, not the microphone.

If you wear a body microphone it will allow you to move more freely, but ensure you wear clothing that allows the microphone to be attached in a suitable position easily. This position is usually towards the centre of the body approximately 18–25 cm (approximately 7–10 inches) below the chin. This can be on a tie, lapel, or suitable dress, shirt, or blouse. You will also need a belt or pocket suitable for the transmitter to be attached to, or placed in. It is also important to avoid scarves and jewelry near the microphone that may interfere with the sound.

If using visual aids, situate your microphone slightly towards the side to which you will be turning in order to avoid diminished sound as your turn your head. Remember that anything you say to anyone will be heard by the group or audience.

If using a body microphone in a classroom setting it is important not to have discussions with teaching assistants or other staff members while the microphone is switched on. Once again remember that anything said to one student will be heard by the whole class.

The teacher as director

Within this role the teacher may be expected to conduct the drama club or produce a drama festival play. Drama classes are, by their very nature, highly participatory and noisy, and therefore they can be very taxing on the voice. To spare the voice, drama classes should be controlled by means of a non-verbal signal, such as a tambourine.

Although the purpose of a drama class is to develop and encourage verbal communication between pupils, at best it also develops co-operative skills. By focusing on interpersonal communication, team work and mutual support, the group can avoid the chaos that results from drama classes that simply expend energy. When a degree of ensemble work develops, the drama class works best and both pupils and teachers enjoy the experience.

It can be helpful and focusing to begin and end a drama class with 'grounding' and calming exercise such as yoga postures, Tai Chi, or simply some still and silent breathing exercises or mirror games. Other teachers will not welcome classes being returned to them in a highly stimulated or over-excited state.

Productions

The inexperienced director would be advised to avoid taking on a full length production in the primary school because these tend to be too long for children to sustain their interest, either as performers or as audience.

When working on a production:

- If possible, avoid calling everyone to rehearsal at the same time. It is better to break the script down into short scenes and rehearse smaller groups. This also reduces the need to discipline large groups.
- Instil a 'professional' work ethic in the cast so that rehearsing can be productive and additional rehearsals are less likely to be necessary. The students are likely to enjoy the structure and benefit from the disciplined approach.
- Ask an experienced colleague to be your assistant director and rehearse crowd scenes while you work with the principal cast.
- Avoid long rehearsals where students are left waiting for their time on stage.
- Appoint a stage management team from the outset as they will shoulder much of the organization and free you for the creative work. There are bound to be experienced members of amateur dramatic groups amongst parents and staff.
- Ensure groups are calmed and focused at the end of drama classes so that they can return to their academic studies in a receptive frame of mind.
- Delegate: involve other departments so that different members of staff can help with music, scenery, and costumes.

Parents find extra rehearsals and long evenings difficult if younger children are involved. It is also important to enlist parental and staff support with regard to organization and assistance, and to delegate from the outset. In primary schools themed programmes, rather than full scale plays, allow participation for a broad range of children, not just the best actors.

Parents do not expect to see 'professional' standards in an elementary or primary school production, and much of the charm lies in the unexpected 'hiccup'. As a general rule, a well rehearsed shorter performance provides an experience that is better for the audience and more positive for the class than an over-ambitious lengthy production.

The teacher as reader/performer

Most teachers find themselves taking on this role as part of their classroom duties. An ability to 'bring words to life' can transform a lesson or lecture. Most teachers read aloud well and enjoy doing so, but a significant number find this is a daunting and often vocally tiring task. There are those who 'feel the throat tighten' as they read and hear a voice produced that they find difficult to recognize as their own; others feel inhibited and self-conscious when having to entertain or be seen to be performing. The close link between performance and teaching is recognized by many and for some, it is an element that they really feel happy to engage in. There are those who are natural communicators and there are those who feel that they did not enter teaching to be 'performers'.

Teachers who are most likely to find themselves in the position of having to read to a class regularly are the kindergarten/pre-primary, infant and primary/elementary school teachers, teachers of English literature and other humanities subjects, and those whose duties include reading at assembly. Teachers of the younger age groups expect to read aloud regularly, but those who find themselves with a younger age group than they trained for are often worried about how effectively they can 'tell the story'. When there is anxiety over reading the voice is likely to become over-used and tired. Some teachers, who qualified through postgraduate schemes reported that their one year course did not provide the advice and practice that they felt they needed to develop expressive sightreading skills.

Educators are knowledgeable about the rudiments of reading and so there is no need to reiterate them here. That there are significant differences between fluent personal reading, and the art and skill of reading aloud to an audience, is not always fully acknowledged. The most important of these differences is that the reader has the book in front of him and can follow the printed word whereas the audience cannot, so they must rely on the voice they hear. The audience is therefore at a considerable disadvantage and must be helped to 'enter the world of the story' through dynamic and expressive interpretation and intelligent phrasing. The art of the teacher who reads to the class is that of the story-teller, an art which, sadly for many children, is being eroded and replaced by technology. In the lives of many children, the primary school teacher is the only adult who ever reads to them. The classroom 'story' takes on enormous importance for children who are not lucky enough to be read to at home. Teachers want to read aloud to the best of their ability, because they want children to be stimulated and excited by words and language, and to be inspired to read avidly for themselves.

The speaker should strive to engage the children's imagination by vocally formulating images of the language. The story is not only contained in the words but in the sound-scape: vowels and consonants add to the music and energy of the language as do alliteration, repetition, pace, inflection, emphasis, and pause. Connecting with and honouring the rhythm gives an added dimension to the story. Most stories offer the reader the opportunity to explore vocal tone and to move away from habitual pitch through characterization. While some may find this challenging, the story is bound to be improved and the characters brought to life more vividly.

Audibility

Speech has to be heard, decoded, and understood before listeners can react to it, so it is important to allow the audience time to go through the listening process. Younger children need to be close to the reader so as to participate in the intimacy of the story. Whatever the age, where possible the class should be brought closer to the speaker to save the voice being overused. This will also improve the chances of reading *to* the group rather than *at* them. Ideally, each child should feel that the story is being read to them personally. If necessary, rearrange the classroom for story time, allowing the group to gather chairs around you or to sit on the floor.

A percentage of children may have undetected hearing issues and, as lip-reading is an important component of the listening process, children should be encouraged to look at the speaker. Both physical and audible information should be given by allowing the face and the body to convey the story, e.g., through eye contact when appropriate. Clarity is enhanced by muscular shaping of the sounds of speech with the lips and tongue. When a reader is committed to the story and to the telling of it, these aspects generally fall into place.

Posture

Even before you speak you are having some effect on the listeners. Whether this effect is positive or negative is dependent on the body language conveyed. At best, the body should be alert but relaxed because any unwanted excess tension will transfer to the voice, so make sure that your chair is comfortable and that you have a glass of water close at hand. The class, too, should be comfortable but should avoid slumping on to desks. Story-telling should be a two-way communication process, with listening being as important as reading or speaking. Younger classes may interrupt and ask questions. Alternatively, a story can be told in a participatory manner by asking the group to react and respond and inviting them to say what they think might be the outcome.

While questions are proof of listening and engagement, when reading to older classes the reader should answer questions concisely and return to the story, or suggest discussing questions at the end. It is important to keep the energy and narrative sustained. As mentioned before, eye contact is needed in order to relate to the listeners. Meaningful phrasing and emphasis of appropriate words helps convey a sense that the story is being told not read.

Eye contact

For some teachers making eye contact while reading is 'easier said than done'. The usual comment is that the teacher is afraid of losing his/her place, which can easily happen in text tightly packed on to the page. When reading anything complicated, such as Dickens or even Mark Twain, the advice is to scan the chapter first and to become familiar with it. If teachers know exactly what they are going to read and when, e.g., if having to read a religious tract at an assembly, the extract should be photocopied and if necessary enlarged. A highlighter can be used to mark words or phrases that signal a pause or an opportunity for the reader to look up. Readers sometimes look up with alarming regularity because they have been led to believe that any eye contact represents good reading practice. They do not make eye contact with intent but rather 'flick' their eyes over the listeners before returning hurriedly to the text. For the listeners, 'looking up' can be annoying if it is done without reason. The golden rule for readers is to look up only when appropriate and to be aware of the whole class, not just a section of it. Eye contact should allow the reader time to include the members of class and allow them time to digest what has just been said. The value for the class lies in being read to by an adult whom they know and can relate to; unless the reader makes contact with the class, they may as well have listened to the radio.

Pace

Most people reading aloud read at a faster pace than they realize. Monitoring the speed at which an individual is reading or speaking is difficult, particularly if the individual is under pressure and does not naturally enjoy the delivery of words. The reader's greatest asset is the ability to allow himself and the audience time. Members of the audience need time to digest one idea before being fed another; they need to be able to hear how one idea develops into the next so that they can build up the progression of ideas and be involved in the development of the narrative. They also need time to 'take on board' new characters, often with unusual names, and to build up, from the language that they hear, a visual image of the action, as well as formulating a response to the incidents and emotions. A slower speech rate also helps the reader because it allows for forward scanning, eye contact, changes of vocal tone for different characters and the building up of an imaginative response to the text; additionally, if readers do not know the story, it allows them to go through their own 'see, decode, understand and react' process. Occasionally, it may be appropriate to repeat a phrase or a word from the text in order to increase the level of the group's involvement.

Scanning ahead

The ability to scan ahead is something that can be improved by practice and confidence. Often it is the panic of losing one's place that prevents an other-wise confident sight-reader from letting the eyes glide over the page. A most useful exercise is to hold a closed book and open it suddenly; let the eyes fall on to a phrase, close the book, look up and speak the phrase. At first the eyes flicker frantically over the page and have to be encouraged to settle on a phrase. If this is done regularly it builds ability and confidence, and is an excellent exercise to do with children from nine years onwards. It begins to extend the eye's peripheral vision and it is this that allows the full sense of a phrase to be taken in and choppy, broken reading improved. It is fun, and it can be practiced first using lists of phrases and idioms because they are less daunting than great blocks of text. Progression can then be made on to more densely blocked text, using books that have larger writing and good spacing.

Suggestions for improving sight-reading

- Ensure your posture is comfortable and aligned so that breathing is free and easy.
- Actively release the shoulders, neck and jaw so that the voice is not constricted.
- Sit or stand with a well aligned and open posture with head, neck, and shoulders relaxed and free so that the voice is capable of effort-less projection.
- If you are not a confident reader, mark your script so that you work out in advance when you can comfortably make eye contact.
- Eye contact allows you to include your audience and share the story, and to read 'to them' not 'at them'.
- Explore the sound-scape and rhythm of the story.

- Employ the aspects of vocal modulation such as pace, pitch, pause, inflection, emphasis, and use the dynamic qualities of vowels and consonants.
- Rehearse character voices.
- If possible rehearse your reading or familiarize yourself with the text.
- Familiarity will allow you to breathe naturally and phrase well so that you are easy to follow and understand.

The teacher as tour guide

Within this role the teacher may be expected to conduct tours to museums and give information on the history of the dinosaur while counting heads, or traipse across ancient battlefields, fighting against the wind and cold, and project the voice while describing the action that took place historically. This role can also include skiing trips, sports tours and a week's educational field trip abroad. In these circumstances, the teacher has to use the voice at high volume for long periods of time in adverse circumstances. As with the field sports teachers, it is important for the teacher to be physically relaxed, warm and hydrated. They should draw the students around them in an orderly group and avoid having to project above the noise of, for example, a busy tourist centre, other tourist groups, an underground train station or the entrance to a busy art gallery. It is important for children to be encouraged always to position themselves in a semi-circle around the teacher so that they can see the teacher and the teacher can see them.

The voice will be spared if the group is divided into sub-groups each with their own adult leader who is responsible for them.

- It can be helpful to dress groups in colour-coded hats, jackets, or sashes for easy identification as this helps with control.
- Some schools divide groups into pairs who must stay together within the group at all times.
- It is important to have a 'control plan' which is rehearsed before the outing, establishing the means by which the group will communi-

cate. This may include flags, whistles or hand signals and can be part of the risk assessment undertaken by the school prior to the outing.

- If the group is allowed to have cell/mobile phones with them, their numbers should be given to the teacher and they should have a number to call should they get lost.
- In order to reduce the need for excessive voice use, a worksheet can be produced for every member of the group, also containing contact information, meeting points and a strategy if the group becomes separated.
- It is important to develop a vocal strategy for use in this role. Too often the teacher resorts to shouting over noise.

Exercises for working outdoors and healthy use of the voice at volume can be found in **Chapter 10**.

The role of music teacher

Within this role the teacher may be expected to be involved in singing classes. For men teaching singing in the primary school, problems can arise because the teacher often has to sing at a pitch far higher than his natural one, which can be both problematic and 'tiring'. Male singing teachers sometimes have difficulty sustaining high pitch for long periods of time, especially those who work with junior schoolchildren or in girls' schools. The use of falsetto is one option but, if in attempting to reach high notes it creates vocal tension, it should be avoided. Instead the note may be suggested through the use of an instrument such as a recorder, piano or pitching fork.

Singing and music teachers, if they are not aware of good positioning at the piano or while bending over seated children playing recorders, may experience postural problems which can lead to voice and back difficulties. Alignment at the piano should be checked; teachers are advised to avoid standing and leaning over to play while at the same time looking up at the class and attempting to sing. This also applies to situations that involve playing while looking backwards at a class. If at all possible, the instrument should be positioned so that it may be used in the best possible ergonomic position.

Teachers should try to 'practice what they preach'. If the class is being told how to breathe, teachers should make sure that they are taking time to breathe well themselves. Children and students should be taught that the breath should be low and deep. Most adults remember choir teachers saying 'Take a big breath' which invariably ends up being a breath that allows far less intake of breath than a breath taken low in the body, using the lower ribs, diaphragm and abdominal muscles. When considering breathing it is important to focus on communication. An aspect of singing that is sometimes neglected is the delivery of the lyrics so that the content is understood and communicated as this will help with phrasing and subsequently improve the breathing.

Points to consider when teaching singing or musical instruments:

- Shoulders should be relaxed when playing the piano, and awkward postures avoided while playing and coaching.
- Posture should be monitored while demonstrating string and wind instruments which can be conducive to shoulder tension, e.g., the physical position for violinists can lead to a forward head and neck position.
- Hydration should be monitored.
- Many music teachers teach in the lunch break and it is important to make sure that rather than rushing from one class into another, teachers take some time out for themselves.
- Rather than speaking or singing over the noise of the class, the teacher should instead first signal for them to stop.
- Teachers should avoid demonstrating to the class when suffering from a cold.

The teacher as consultant

Most teachers are expected to take part in parent evenings. Apart from the pressures of meeting parents and discussing sometimes sensitive issues, this can be a stressful occasion because it almost always follows on after a full day's teaching. Most parents, while concerned about their children, are appreciative of what is done by teachers and are generally good-natured but occasionally, they can be defensive or even aggressive. Although assaults are uncommon, the pressure on the teacher is enormous and the effect on an already tired and stressed individual is considerable.

The most vocally challenging situation for teachers is when more than one teacher shares the same space for consultations, because this increases the ambient noise level. An additional noise can be the regular bells or buzzers sounded to signal the next appointment.

To lessen the pressure on the teacher and protect the voice the following strategies are proposed:

- If possible make sure that there is time to have a proper break between the usual working day and the timetabled parent consultations.
- It is important for teachers to keep well hydrated throughout the evening.
- Ideally, tea breaks should be scheduled into an evening of consultations.
- Seating should be comfortable. Straining over the table while talking should be avoided.
- Head and shoulder position should be checked and monitored throughout the evening.
- Chairs should be well positioned so that there is no need for the teacher to raise his or her voice when talking to parents.
- The consultation should be planned so that opening and closing statements are available to signal clearly that the consultation is over. Standing up and offering a hand will also signal that the interview is over.

Newly qualified teachers

Consultation sessions can be daunting and newly qualified teachers should not hesitate to ask colleagues for help in giving honest feedback. Alternatively, an educational consultant or experienced member of staff could offer a training session to all new students or the entire school. Helpful training sessions may include negotiation strategies and conflict resolution.

Pastoral care

If a teacher is required to undertake a pastoral care role, it is important to voice their feelings should they feel uncomfortable or out of their depth, and to ask for support and training. It is not unreasonable to ask for conflict resolution training, help in managing difficult situations, and identifying and responding to worrying social and family situations. Many schools now have trained counsellors who can be consulted when appropriate.

The supply or agency teacher

'Supply' is a role that teachers take on for a variety of reasons including returning to teaching after a period away, wanting freelance employment while raising a family, and looking for short-term post-retirement work. Others may have moved from one area to another and may choose to experience a variety of schools in the new area before applying for a permanent post. They may be teachers who do not want a permanent position, or teachers who have found the administrative workload too much and simply want to be able to do what they were trained for and teach without the additional pressures of marking homework and organization. Whatever the reason, there are a number of specific demands made on the teacher in this role.

The employment of supply teachers has increased enormously over recent years. They not only step into the breach when staff members are sick but also provide cover so that teachers have free time for administrative work and planning, and to allow full-time staff to undertake continuing development training. They frequently fill the gaps that occur between permanent staff leaving and new appointments being made. It appears to be a workforce that is growing as stress in schools increases, resulting in greater levels of absenteeism. As such they form an important section of the teaching community but one that at present receives little support or training.

The UK is not the only country where supply teachers are increasingly important as similar situations occur in many other countries, although the systems they employ may differ.

Potential vocal issues

Supply teachers encounter vocal difficulties as a result of the variable nature of their work. It would be wrong to presume that all supply teachers will encounter problems; there will be many who have had years of successful teaching and whose training has included a solid grounding in voice work, but for some this is not the case:

- A number of teachers who immigrate to the UK choose to supply teach in the first instance. Working within an alien environment and learning the workings of another education system is both challenging and tiring.
- For some, English may be a second language and this in itself may produce added stress and anxiety about being understood.
- The teacher who does not teach on a regular basis is less likely to build vocal stamina steadily over a number of weeks and therefore, may be more susceptible to vocal problems.
- Lack of stamina can present as a problem when teachers suddenly encounter a noisy class or find themselves teaching a week of physical education.
- Some find a sporadic work pattern better for their voices because they do not need to accept a job if their voice is tired.
- Discipline can be difficult because the students know that the teacher will not be around for long, so they will probably not be challenged about their behaviour. This may result in the class becoming noisier

than usual and the teacher using high volume or finding it necessary to shout.

- There are additional strains on the supply teacher that may lead to an increased likelihood of vocal stress or ill health. In many primary schools, supply teachers are expected to stay at school and mark the day's work before they leave. This can result in a very long day and can become exhausting if the teacher works every day.

- The supply teacher meets a new set of students and a new set of 'germs' several times a week, so they may be more susceptible to infection and more likely to suffer voice loss.

- All these pressures and confusions create tension and undoubtedly place demands on the vocal health and confidence of the teacher.

A constantly changing challenge

A major cause of difficulty for supply teachers is that they are always entering an 'unknown zone'. Not being in familiar surroundings is stressful in itself, and additional pressure comes from not being able to relate to other members of staff. They are constantly negotiating new student–teacher relationships as well as meeting new colleagues and being 'outsiders' in an unknown situation. Some report they are not properly met and introduced to colleagues, or given essential information. There can be confusion as to which classes will be taught by the supply teacher; this leads to delays at the start of the class and in turn, breaks the sense of 'normality' for the students. Some students see supply teachers as an 'easy target' and take the opportunity to 'have some fun' at their expense by pranks such as swapping names or inventing new ones when asked who they are. Others give incorrect directions as to the whereabouts of classes in order to confuse the supply teacher and make them late. Students have been known to state 'I don't do work for supply teachers' when asked to get on with their task.

Common problems encountered by supply teachers

- Not all schools provide the supply teacher with enough information, such as clear directions to the school, maps of the layout of the school, catering facilities, and toilets.
- Classrooms often lack adequate essential materials such as fresh and working felt-tip pens for the white boards.
- Sometimes, instructions are not given clearly or correctly so that the teacher may have prepared one lesson and then suddenly have to change the content and work without proper preparation.
- Work set by the class teacher may not have been left out in a place where it is easily visible, leading to delay and a loss of class focus.
- The teacher may not be familiar with the subject at all – this can be particularly difficult when a subject requires specialized knowledge such as mathematics, a foreign language, or science. Equally daunting and vocally demanding are subjects such as drama, or physical education, or games.
- Even if the supply teacher has previously taught the subject, it may be necessary to adapt to a very different way of approaching it. Help in doing so may not be easy to find because of pressure of work on the permanent staff.
- A complaint from supply teachers is that, as a result of poor organization on the part of the school, or bad behaviour in the class, they do not teach but 'caretake'. This can be professionally frustrating and demoralizing.
- Supply teachers sometimes find themselves working with the same class for a longer period of time if the need arises. Although they are then able to bond with the class, some teachers find that the parents do not take them seriously, especially if the teacher needs to discipline the child.
- Supply teachers are by their very existence a 'second best' option. The class is always better catered for by a permanent teacher with shared experience and knowledge of the students. If a class is continuously

being presented with temporary staff their work will suffer, and they know this and feel neglected.

Other problems for the supply teacher are more personally specific:

- The teacher may not be local and may have to travel a considerable distance to get to the school. This may mean that they are often tired especially if they have taught at several different schools in one week.
- The teacher may leave home much earlier than is necessary in order to negotiate new routes and unknown distances.
- Agencies ring round teachers on their list once the need becomes apparent at the start of the school day. This means that teachers relying on supply work must be ready to teach every day, although they may not get work. Alternatively, they may receive a late summons and be ill-prepared and have to rush around at the last moment, arriving at the school tense and flustered.
- The teacher may be returning to teaching after a break and so confidence may be low. The effects of low self-esteem and a sense of not belonging may impact on posture and breath.
- The career supply teacher does not have a salary to rely on and is dependent on working as often as possible in order to earn a living. They know that they have long periods out of work during the school holidays and so are often reluctant to refuse work when it is offered. This means that they are more likely to teach when they are not well, and when they would take a day off if they were permanently employed.

The supply teacher is increasingly a crucial member of the teaching profession. The job is a difficult and demanding one and requires flexibility and confidence. As supply teachers are not on a school's permanent staff roll, it is often difficult for them to access ongoing training in order for them to respond to the changing curriculum and to serve the students as best they can.

The many different roles assumed by supply teachers are possible only because of their flexibility and ability to respond to the demands that the profession makes on them.

Suggestions for establishing presence and protecting the voice

- On the way to the school in the car, or even on public transport, warm up by releasing shoulders, neck, and jaw by yawning, stretching the tongue, and humming.
- Make a positive entrance: walk into an unknown classroom with confident body language.
- Hold the space physically by avoiding shuffling the feet, making confident eye contact and using a commanding but friendly vocal tone.
- Prepare a 'ready lesson' that is easily adaptable to any class, in case work has not been set.

The many roles of the teacher

There will always be aspects of a job that appeal to some people while others dislike them. In taking on these auxiliary duties, personality is a significant factor; some may feel happy to teach 10-year-old 'tearaways' but are daunted by their parents. Some teachers enter the profession because they enjoy performance and role play. There is a significant skills crossover between teachers, actors, lawyers and the clergy; all demand an element of performance and verbal skill. Many teachers enjoy the performance element of teaching. Others have a passion to teach but hate to perform and feel very strongly that, when they entered the profession, these peripheral demands were never made clear to them. Unfortunately, without the willingness to carry out at least some of these duties effectively, career prospects may be limited. One way of surmounting the problem is for teachers to remain resolute if asked to undertake a commitment that they do not feel comfortable with, and to offer to do something else instead, although this is not to underestimate how difficult it can be to withstand persuasion.

Chapter outline

- The teacher as orator
- The teacher as sports coach
- The teacher as entertainer
- Microphone technique
- The teacher as director
- Productions
- The teacher as reader and performer
- The teacher as tour guide
- The role of music teacher
- The teacher as consultant
- Pastoral care
- Newly qualified teachers
- The supply or agency teacher
- Potential vocal issues
- A constantly changing challenge
- Common problems encountered by supply teachers
- Suggestions for establishing presence and protecting the voice
- The many roles of the teacher

References and further reading

Atkinson A. 2008. *Speech–Making and Presentation Made Easy.* London: Vermillion.

Leith S. 2012. *You Talkin' to Me?* London: Profile Books.

Toastmasters International. Available at: <https://www.toastmasters.org/> [Accessed August 2017].

10

Being heard

The following chapters offer a variety of exercises that have a broad application to all professional voice users. Some will, by their nature, be more appropriate to class situations but many offer a firm foundation for general voice use. The exercises aim to establish an integrated physical and vocal approach. Some exercises are for specific muscles; others offer a planned sequence of exercises or routines for the voice. Regular periods of exercise are preferable to occasional long sessions and therefore, these routines are designed to last for between 10 and 20 minutes. You may notice some repetition of exercises within different routines. This is to allow readers to work through a sequence without needing to locate preparatory exercises elsewhere.

The exercises raise awareness of habitually held tension in muscles, establish low placement of the breath, and encourage efficient use of energy in body and voice. Habits of any sort are difficult to change and often develop out of the individual's personality and reaction to situations; this makes it difficult for the individual to be objective about where and how tension is held, so working with another person can be helpful. The way in which people like to work is also highly individual; in recognition of this, we have included a variety of approaches so that if one approach does not appeal, another may. If the vocal problem is a recurring one, we would strongly advise seeking professional help before starting on an exercise plan. These exercises will help maintain a healthy voice and prevent problems caused by inappropriate breathing and physical alignment, but they should never be seen as a substitute for voice therapy if that is required. The participative value of voice work within the classroom has already been stressed, so we have also included exercises that can be done with school and college classes. With a little imagination exercises can be adapted to suit all ages.

Readers will note a change in the writing style in the three remaining chapters of the book. This has been done in order to address the reader directly and make the exercises both more accessible and easier to follow.

Audibility, volume, projection, clarity, and working in open spaces

For a significant number of educators, audibility and clarity is a problem. Being audible means you can be heard but for those involved in education, audibility is not enough. Being clear and understandable is essential. If you cannot be heard the message is lost and your status is undermined. Classrooms are not always built with acoustics in mind, and many educators find working in halls and open spaces particularly taxing. Clarity is a complex issue often related to a lack of volume, but low volume is not always the culprit. It is likely that a number of contributing factors, such as tension, low morale, poor breath support, a lack of resonance, too high or too low a pitch, and diction are involved. Class management and poor communication should also be assessed and if necessary, improved.

It is essential to understand how body language can lead to negative perceptions as well as reducing the ability to project. It is also important to remember that personality, and not just voice, should be projected and that this in turn will create a greater impact on an audience.

Changing habits

If your habitual voice use has been quiet, a louder sound might feel overbearing or simply unnatural. It is important to be able to use the voice to achieve your goals, and this may mean developing new styles of vocal use. You should strive to attempt to adjust your volume slightly when meeting new people, when shopping, and in the home.

When working on volume and when addressing volume-related issues in the classroom, remember that work on volume is most effective:

- with confident and open posture;
- with sufficient breath control and support;
- with a relaxed and stress-free approach that does not lead to forcing the voice or shouting;
- with an ability to release and sustain breath rather than to force it out of the body;
- with an understanding of the relationship between energy and breath: energy should not be seen as leading to restrictive tension;
- with an ability to remove focus from the larynx, using breath and energy to produce increased volume, not increased laryngeal effort;
- when increasing the use of range and clarity for emphasis rather than simply relying on volume;
- with the use of a slower pace and the effective use of pause;
- when increasing articulatory precision;
- when working on the entire pitch range rather than on a narrow, limited range;
- with fine control of a subtle range of sound rather than the extremes of whisper and shout; and
- with an awareness of the link between sung and spoken voice in order to develop a sense of flow.

When working on volume and when addressing volume-related issues in the classroom, remember that work on volume is of limited effectiveness:

- if working on volume without prior work on relaxation, posture, and alignment;
- if the voice is forced and without sufficient breath support, often resulting in a breathy, unfocused sound;
- when voicing under pressure to increase volume rather than using resonance to increase the amount of sound created;

245

- when speaking *at* rather than *to* people: not using direct eye contact and appropriate body posture to aid communication;
- when using too much stress and not enough inflection to emphasize and deliver the message;
- with exaggerated body posture, for example, head jutting forward, finger pointing and jabbing, and a forward thrust to the body; or
- if the voice is monotonous and uses a narrow range with a subsequent lack of variety in delivery.

Common errors

In an attempt to create clarity by creating additional volume, many teachers opt for what they consider the obvious solution – they shout in an unhealthy manner with the following outcomes:

- Good alignment is lost, shoulders are raised, and breathing shifts to the upper chest.
- The head is thrust forward and the jaw is clenched. Instead of creating more sound the voice becomes locked and strangulated.
- Those with naturally quiet voices may find themselves not necessarily shouting but 'pushing and squeezing' the voice out, resulting in a hard, 'thin' tone which may be perceived as unfriendly, fearful, tentative, or ungenerous.
- A 'hard onset' is produced when initiating a note. It is important to safeguard the voice by synchronizing breath with the approximation of the vocal folds.

Adjust your focus

Focusing on the needs of the class or audience is critical, and can help reduce tension by removing the focus from oneself. Consider these class or audience needs. They need to:

- hear you and engage with the speaker;
- feel that the speaker is relaxed and in control, without 'feeling anxious' about them;

- have the speaker make eye contact with them and speak 'to' them not 'at' them;
- feel the speaker's commitment and passion;
- hear the clearly articulated information at a reasonable rate that allows them time to decode and digest the message; and
- be able to absorb more information when the delivery has an interesting and energized 'vocal tone and verbal colour'.

Projection is therefore not just about volume: it also requires you to engage with and enthuse the audience with your passion.

Posture and alignment

We have spoken at length about the importance of posture and head position, and of the freedom needed in the muscles of the shoulders, neck, and jaw. This advice is even more critical when increasing volume. The instinctive energy recruited when organizing large groups and involving any element of crowd control or discipline, works against the idea of a free neck. Many educators find themselves using pointing and even prodding gestures with the fingers and head in addition to speech. When this happens, it is no surprise that not only the power in the voice is lost but also, the control of the class.

The value of stillness cannot be emphasized enough (by stillness we mean free, grounded stillness, not rigid, held stillness) but also, the quietness and stillness required to allow easy breathing and clear thinking. A quality of quiet, still control is generally afforded high status.

There are many misconceptions about making the voice easily audible which work against good posture and calm control. The language used to encourage better audibility tends to produce images of the voice 'pushing' forward. We hear 'Speak up', 'Speak out', 'Throw the voice', 'Project the voice', 'Reach the back of the room', 'Notch up the volume', and even 'Hit them with the sound'. In reality such suggestions only add to the lecturer's or teacher's tension and to misuse of energy. It is much better, and of course more appropriate, to suggest that the whole class is 'Included in the conversation' or that the 'Information is shared', thus concentrating on the intention behind the word and conveying this rather than simply creating more sound.

When told to 'speak up' most people simply raise their pitch and become strident, which is very stressful both for the speaker and the listeners. A voice that is shrill is alienating rather than engaging or inclusive. The effort involved in pushing the sound out is the very thing that limits it. If this style of delivery becomes habitual the voice is likely to become uncomfortable and ultimately may suffer damage.

For this reason and for the sake of effective communication, avoid responding when angry or frustrated. A voice that is perceived to be 'out of control' has low status and suggests desperation or intimidation. A projected voice should never be shrill, strident or perceived as 'bad tempered'. It is often much more effective to pause, and take time to adjust your alignment and raise your status, before responding in a calm, controlled and 'grounded' manner.

'Grounding' the body and voice

'Grounding' is associated with establishing a sense of weight in the lower body, and developing a feeling of a low centre of gravity, through connecting with the ground/floor rather than holding tension in the upper body. When this is well established it is easier to release the upper body, engage the low abdominal muscles and produce a breath supported vocal tone. Try this exercise:

1. Facing a partner, stand approximately one metre apart.
2. Both raise arms to shoulder height. Place your hands against your partner's hands with palms touching.
3. Leaning forward, begin to mutually support each other's weight.
4. Notice that it is easier to connect with the low breath muscles when you feel weight in the lower body. In this position call 'Follow this way!' to someone behind you..

Now repeat the exercise against a wall instead of with a partner. Give your full weight 'to' the wall. This position will also open the chest. Connect with the breath muscles on a /hoh/ sound and then call again to someone behind you, saying, 'Follow this way!' Repeat several times getting louder each time. Once you have done this try to stand and feel the same sense of weight in the body. Repeat the /hoh/ sound several times, again getting louder each time.

Skillful projection of the voice allows the speaker to be heard in large spaces without amplification. It requires range, clear articulation, and a desire not only to take physical command of the space but to share the information with the audience. Successful projection is dependent on the ability to provide an adequate, unrestricted breath supply to fully support free vocal fold movement. A well supported, free and unrestricted note will allow specific resonators to give warmth, energy and volume to the voice. The fear involved in addressing large groups of people is likely to mitigate a relaxed, well supported sound, so creating a vicious circle. It is often better to address underlying confidence issues before attempting to approach them technically but sometimes, working on volume helps to overcome the fear by altering the relationship between the teacher and the class or the lecturer and the audience.

Exercises to help 'free' the sound from tension

1. **Smiling.** Smiling with the face and eyes, and feeling the lift in the soft palate before you begin to voice, is advisable. This can be practiced if you imagine singing a very high note but staying silent: simply adopt the smile posture. Experience the sensation of the open pharynx with lifted soft palate, and space behind the tongue and in the mouth.

2. **Silent laughing.** With hands firmly holding round the waist (thumbs at the back, fingers round the front) laugh silently on the sounds /hoh/hoh/hoh/. (Feel the sense of space behind the tongue.)

3. **Singing.** Choose a simple line from a song and with a partner, take it in turns to exaggerate the quality and length of the vowels and the pitch range. Notice how there is more demand on the breath, range and resonance. Never push the sound, even playfully. If you find this difficult try using only the sound /lah/ lah/lah/.

4. **Shaking out.** Release the sounds /yoh/ /yah/ /noh/ /nah/ /woh/ /wah/ while vigorously shaking the body. Sustain the initial /y/ /n/ and /w/ before releasing into the vowel sound. Starting at the feet, shake out again, allowing the sound to travel up through the body. With the weight on both feet, release the knees; gently bounce and shake out. Keep the jaw and the tongue loose and the soft palate lifted (use an open-mouthed smile to lift the soft palate). Repeat the same series of sounds, and starting quietly, build the volume.

Keep the sense of openness in the throat and avoid 'throwing back the head' or 'locking the neck'.

Creating more sound

It is important to understand that in order to amplify sound, what is needed is space in the mouth and oropharynx for amplification, and breath to initiate the note and carry the sound forward into the mask of the face to create resonance and clarity.

Four quick exercises for creating oral space

1. In order to create more space in the mouth, which is the most movable resonator, stroke the jaw down with hands on both sides of the face and feel the added space between the molars at the back of the mouth.

2. Stretch the tongue as far as you can out of the mouth and hold it there for a few seconds, then slowly release it and allow it to return to a relaxed position touching the lower front and side teeth. Let the jaw remain loose.

3. Keeping the lips sealed, create maximum space in the mouth as you move the upper and lower molars away from each other.

4. Yawn freely and feel the size of the cavity you create. You may feel this more if you keep your lips together as you yawn.

Four quick exercises for developing breath support

1. With lips rounded, blow gently onto your hand in a sustained manner. Place the other hand below the navel. Allow the muscles below the navel to move towards the spine as the breath is expelled.

2. Repeat the above exercise but much more slowly and with less pressure.

3. Imagine you have a large cake in front of you. Blow out 10 candles in a sustained manner while monitoring the breathing muscles below the navel.

4. Repeat the exercise but voice the sound /moo/ each time you blow out a candle. The sounds /mah/ /may/ and /maw/ can also be used.

Four quick exercises for smooth onset

1. Create an 'inside smile' as if you were smiling with the muscles in the back of the mouth in the area of the molars and uvula. You should feel as if you are about to initiate a yawn. You will become aware of the space at the back of your tongue and your lifted soft palate; holding this position, gently sound the word *hoe* and then drop the /h/ and gently sound the word *owe*.

2. Being very aware of the space at the back of your tongue and your lifted soft palate, place /h/ before the following words: *eel, ale, own, I, all, it, ear*, so you say: /h/eel, /h/ale, /h/own, /h/i, /h/all, /h/it, /h/ear.

3. Once this has been achieved, omit the /h/ and maintaining the space at the back of the tongue and with a lifted soft palate, repeat the words without the /h/. Envisage the action of /h/ but do not form it.

4. Being aware of the need to 'glide' onto vowels and avoid a glottal onset, formulate sentences containing words beginning with vowels such as: 'Andrew often asks for ice-cream but Owen only offers oranges'.

Four quick exercises for forward placement

1. Using the word *yum*, sustain the /m/ sound and placing your hands lightly on your face feel the vibrations on your lips and in the mask of the face. Avoid pinching the lips together and create as much space as you can in the mouth as you make the sound.

2. Imagine you are eating something very tasty and using the words 'very nice', explore the vibrations in the /v/ and /n/ sounds. You should feel these in the mask of the face and the nose.

3. Using the sounds /b/ and /p/, explode the sounds as if you were blowing 'darts' at a target. You can feel this 'pressure' on your hand if you put it a few inches away from your mouth as you produce the sounds.

4. Block your nose with your fingers and say: *Why did David Briar dig up those poppies today?* Use the tip of the tongue to flick the /d/ sound forward and the lips to propel the /p/ and /b/ sounds. To test the difference between forward and backward placement, repeat the exercise speaking the line through the nose, then again without any nasal quality to the sounds. Repeat several times, extending the vowels in 'why', 'David', and 'today', increasing the volume each time.

More exercises for forward placement

Test your placement by positioning your fingers over your nose and speaking this exercise:

/b/ /b/ /b/ /bah/

/g/ /g/ /g/ /gah/

The sound should be completely forward and free and should not enter the nose at all. If it does, it indicates tension in the tongue, soft palate or back of the throat.

Now speak a phrase. It is important to choose a phrase that does not contain the nasal sounds /m/ /n/ /ng/; the following are useful:

This is the house that Jack built.
Workers built the old wall by the field.

The path through the woods is used by walkers.

How sorry he was to see her go.

Carla Jacoby hiked up the hill to view the valley below.

Put your books away please class!

Quiet please everybody!

Ready, steady, GO!

Over here class.

The art of projection: some pointers from actors

It might be helpful to consider the way in which actors develop the art of projection. Actors are required to project over distance and therefore, they learn strategies that can prove useful to professional voice users. Theatres vary in size from an intimate 60- to a vast 1000-seater auditorium.

Actors, often excellent communicators off stage as well as on, do not rely only on high volume in order to be heard. An actor who is comfortable in a very large space has learned how resonance gives body and carrying power to the voice, and how keeping the 'thought' and intention behind the words at all times adds to clear delivery and audibility. Actors speak with a character's desire and commitment to change another character's opinion, to alter a situation or achieve a goal and the term 'motivation' is used in this process. It is very common for the meaning of a phrase to be lost to an audience if the actor has lost concentration on the thought and the intention behind the words. Likewise, teachers, lecturers or trainers who do not feel a natural enthusiasm for the subject, or who feel coerced into teaching a subject that they would rather not teach, can develop audibility problems because they have limited commitment to the words.

Actors learn through experience that at times it is important to allow slight pauses before important words and phrases in order to allow them to stand out, and that intensity of feeling and commitment can aid audibility. Physical stillness and a low intense vocal volume are often used for the most significant of speeches which, despite the low volume, can still be heard clearly. Learning to rely on lower volume while increasing muscularity takes experience and confidence. An expressive voice uses more intonation, range and vocal colour, and all these qualities increase the ability of an audience to hear and understand.

Consonants

In addition, actors are concerned with the energized use of consonants, particularly the final ones that define words. An example of this is the difference between the words *road, rogue, roam, rose'*, and *rope*, or *laugh, lark, large, lard, last,* when spoken. The definition of the last consonant is needed if the word is going to be heard and understood, otherwise confusion can occur when final consonants are ill-defined. Speech is made up of voiced and voiceless sounds. In large spaces it is the voiced sounds that carry because they set up vibrations in the space. Voiceless consonants need even more accuracy and precision, because they do not have the vibration to help them carry.

The connection that consonants have with meaning has been discussed in Chapter 7. Their function as a means of assisting audibility over distance is quite specific. Over half the consonants are voiced, e.g., /b/ is voiced whereas /p/ is created only with breath, /d/ is voiced and /t/ is created only with breath. Examples of other voiced sounds are /m/ /ng/ /n/ /l/ /r/ /z/. As voiced sounds, these consonants create vibration and resonance and so enhance audibility. If speakers engage with the consonants they commit to them in terms of breath and muscle, and this too develops the volume. By committing to the word, there is a greater muscularity in the mask of the face, so the voice is placed forward and is therefore more audible. There is also a perception of status and confidence produced by firm, committed consonants and the resonance that they produce which, along with easier lip-reading from the audience or class, enhances the speaker's chances of being heard. When speech has lost its spontaneity and become automatic, or when the speaker is not committed to the content of the language nor the desire to communicate it, elision of consonant clusters and de-voicing of voiced sounds are much more likely to occur, resulting in dull and inaudible speech.

Exercises for consonants

These exercises can be done with classes of any age.

1. Try to explore the dynamic in the initial consonant of the following words beginning with the consonant /b/. Notice how the breath gathers behind the muscles in the mask of the face, behind the lips. Build up the pressure before exploding the sound through on the following words, using as much physical movement and energy as you can:

   burst   bubble   bounce   bound.

2. In the same way explore the dynamic of /d/ when saying the following words:

   dash   direct   destroy   daub.

3. Explore the dynamic of /g/ when saying the following words:

   giggle   gash   grapple   gush.

4. Explore the dynamic of /n/ when saying the following words:

   niggle   nuzzle   nimble   nudge.

5. Explore the dynamic of /z/ in different positions within the words when saying:

   zoom   ooze   lazy   zebra   fizz.

6. Imagine that you are playing tennis and 'bat' consonants over the net with energy, using good breath support and experiencing the build up and release of the breath on the initial consonant.

7. Once you have done that, create a 'tennis match' using two people to serve and return words that begin with consonants, exploring light and flexible sound and movement as well as the forceful dynamic, e.g:

ball	*bash*	*bounce*
dive	*delve*	*dash*
gird	*glide*	*glimmer*
move	*murmur*	*mumble*
lash	*lob*	*limp.*

8.   Work on difficult consonant combinations to exercise and make demands on the flexibility and agility of the articulators. Here are some examples:

> *sixth form* (which is often reduced to *sick form*);
> *fifth* (which often becomes *fif*);
> *text* (which often becomes *tex*);
> *precinct* (which often becomes *precing*);
> *subject* (which often becomes *subjec*).

In British English when an /s/ (a voiceless sound) follows a voiced consonant, it is generally spoken as a voiced /z/. To experience this, speak the following words first with the spelled yet voiceless /s/ and then with the spoken voiced /s/ (pronounced /z/ in the place of the spelled /s/). Notice the difference that the resonance in the voiced sound makes. We do not use these strongly voiced consonants in close conversation but they are necessary in larger spaces or when speaking to larger groups:

eyes	*ears*	*hands*	*faces*
has	*is*	*was*	*his*
hers	*knees*	*ideas*	*calls*
pens	*roads*	*seas*	*easy*

Now try:

> *Friends, Romans, countrymen, lend me your ears;*
> *I come to bury Caesar, not to praise him.*

From: William Shakespeare, Julius Caesar, Act III, scene ii.

Other examples of the frequency of a voiced /z/ for the spelt /s/ are:

houses	*gardens*	*churches*	*fields*
onions	*apples*	*oranges*	*bananas*
planes	*trains*	*cars*	*bicycles*
horses	*lambs*	*crows*	*cows*
vans	*tractors*	*diggers*	*lorries*

halls   houses   buildings mountains
schools   bags   pencils   rulers

Compare these with the spoken and written /s/ which follows a voiceless consonant:

bikes   reefs   lights   ropes

Try saying these words with a final /z/ and notice how awkward it feels.

Further exercises for muscularity and clarity of speech can be found in Chapter 11.

Vowels

All vowels are voiced and can significantly help the carrying power and musicality of the voice but in contemporary speech, we tend to undervalue the vowels and do not give them their full length or energy. Some people perceive those who commit fully to vowels to be flamboyant and extrovert, personality traits that we shy away from. This is unfortunate because vowels also carry enormous musical and emotional value and if used fully, give both resonance and range to the voice while at the same time increasing flow and contributing to audibility.

Over-articulation of vowels and consonants in small spaces or close proximity to pupils, students or colleagues can be deemed overbearing, aggressive, and socially inappropriate.

Exercises for vowels

1. The vowel in soon is /oo/. Speak this vowel only and over-extend its length and musicality.

2. Repeat this exercise with the word 'swarm' extending the length of the vowel /aw/.

3. Isolate the vowels in the following words and string them together in an extended manner, without the intrusion of any consonants:

    How sweet the moonlight sleeps upon this bank!
    From: William Shakespeare, *The Merchant of Venice*, Act V, scene i.

The resulting sound will be heard as: /ow/ /ee/ /u / /oo/ /ai/ /ee/ /u/ /o/ /i/ /a/.

In everyday speech vowels can become clipped and lose their resonant properties. When speaking over distance it is important to use the resonance and spatial quality of vowels to enhance their innate carrying power.

Developing resonance

When a voice is resonant, it is more likely to be vibrant, engaging, and therefore have more carrying power. Many people are unaware of their own resonance but it is easy to feel the vibrations in the mask of the face, the head, and the chest.

1.   Gently tap on the mask of the face while humming on /m/ /n/ /ng/ /v/ and /z/. Be aware of the vibrations around the nose, on the forehead, the skull and on the lips. Vibrations can also be felt on the back of the neck.

2.   Beat the chest with a fist, while sounding /mah/ and /maw/ as this will connect you to your chest resonance.

3.   Opening out from consonants /m/ /n/, /ng/, /v/ and /z/ to vowels /oh/, /aw/, /ay/ and /ah/ will transfer the resonance to the vowels.

4.   Using the phrases *many many mumbling men, rumbling volcanoes, Zoe is a zebra at the zoo*, and *murmuring music*, explore and enjoy the resonance you create when intoning. Exaggerate and enjoy the vibrations.

5.   Feel the resonance in the vowels and consonants in this phrase: *Divide yourselves into teams, please.* Pay special attention to the vibrations in the highlighted sounds: *Divide **yourselves into teams, please.***

Those with very resonant voices need to balance sound with muscular diction in order to ensure they can be clearly understood.

Varying the pitch

Explore other pitches. We often use the same limited pitch range habitually and do not realize the full variety of pitch that is open to us. When attempting to be heard over distance, a common error is to keep the voice on one pitch. Before using your voice over distance try the following:

Using the phrase *Gather around please*, explore your vocal choices by:

- laughing as you speak (if this is difficult and unnatural use a 'ho ho' mock laugh);
- singing the phrase;
- calling the line;
- beating the chest as you speak;
- speaking each word on a different pitch;
- slurring the line as if you were drunk;
- speaking it in slow motion; and
- starting as low as you can, let the voice rise in pitch for *around* and drop down again for *please*.

When you find the innate musical and emotional value of the vowels you will also tap into the greater vocal resonance of your voice. Notice the way the vowel sounds carry; because they are voiced and continuing, they have vocal 'body'. If time is taken and overly clipped speech is avoided with more balance between consonants and vowel sounds, it is possible to develop a greater ability to fill the space easily. Sometimes this can be achieved by simply slowing down.

Exploring volume

With all of the following exercises it is essential to monitor breath capacity, control and support. A common fault is the tendency to let too much air 'escape' initially, causing a sudden rather than a gradual decrease in the size of the ribcage.

The following exercises require a playful approach:

1. Using the sound /sh/, imitate the sound of the sea ebbing and flow-ing. As the wave breaks on the sea shore, increase the volume and reduce it as the sea ebbs away: /sh . . . SH/ . . . /sh . . . SH/ . . . /sh . . . SH/.

2. Using the sounds /v/ or /ng/, imitate the sound of a car or a plane approaching, passing, and receding.

3. Using the sound /z/, imitate the noise of a mosquito approaching, passing, receding, and returning /zzzzzzzz/. Similar exercises (such as approaching and departing chugging trains, and soft and loud ringing or tolling bells), may be tried using sung or chanted, rather than spoken, sounds.

4. Imagine playing with the volume control on a radio and try to imi-tate the variety of sound. Work with the sounds /woh/, /wee/, /wow/ either on their own or as a blend. For all these exercises a variety of pitch should be achieved.

5. Making sure posture is maintained, imagine a line of sound that is some small distance away, say two metres (6 feet 9 inches). Try to pull in this line smoothly, increasing volume as the line draws closer. This concept of drawing in prevents the common problem of a head thrust in an attempt to increase volume. Use the sound /hah/ initially to avoid hard attack. Any phrase or sentence may be used to develop this exercise.

6. With the image of the radio volume control in exercise 4, use the sentence *Good evening this is the ten o'clock news* to alter the volume spontaneously. Avoid excessive loudness but do encourage a subtle range of sound. Working in pairs, A 'conducts' B through increasing and decreasing levels of volume, while B speaks a known passage such as a poem, a nursery rhyme or any piece of text. If B is unable to recall such a passage, the alphabet, months of the year, days of the week, or even counting can be used.

7. Determine the point of focus for a sound some distance away but not too far for easy delivery. Imagine rolling a light 'ball of sound'

across the floor to the target. Use an underarm bowling movement to follow the sound through. Use /moh/ /mah/ and /may/, increasing the volume as the sound rolls to its destination. This exercise may be extended by using short sentences, but these should contain continuants and not plosives to encourage continuity. Care must be taken to avoid the glottal stop between vowels. Initially, increase volume gradually on each word, then increase volume phrase by phrase. The following short phrases may be useful:

> *Over every ocean, over every hill the old eagle flew.*
> *Hour after hour after hour, after hour.*
> *Again and again and again all afternoon and into the evening.*
> *Throw the oranges to Oscar please Alex.*
> *I am anxious to avoid arguing with Ernest and Andrew.*

Intention and definition

In the theatre, what audiences often consider inaudible is in fact perfectly loud. What it lacks, more often than not, is clear intention and definition of thought. These are aspects that educators can work on, and which will improve delivery and therefore audibility immediately. Anyone working too hard to produce a louder volume is likely to 'lock' breath and neck, thus reducing peripheral vision, raising the pitch and giving an impression of aggression that may lead to a loss of goodwill and attention from the class/group/audience.

When working with actors it becomes apparent that the loudest volumes (which are not used all that often by actors and certainly not for prolonged periods) are sustainable with less effort when coming from a free and open body position and appropriate breath support. The minute the neck locks, high volume without vocal discomfort is not an option. The actor works to find ways of producing volume without 'closing down' the open neck position. Above all, the actor fills the space physically and vocally without 'pushing' to reach the back. Most actors work to develop an omnidirectional approach because so many theatres today are not built with a proscenium arch and the audience is often seated behind, as well as in front of them. An actor–audience relationship is not unlike that of the educator who, it is said, 'needs eyes in the back of the head'. This omnidirectional approach involves:

- keeping an active level of communication going all the time;
- developing peripheral vision;
- using voice that is resonant and therefore has carrying power;
- using defined consonants; and
- receiving as well as emitting energy.

In terms of the space itself, it is important to perceive it as being inhabited by the class/group or audience, as well as by the educator or actor. There should never be an 'us and them' approach because this is likely to promote a feeling of alienation. Actors usually walk about the space before their performance in order to familiarize themselves with it and to find out how their voices behave within the space. Once they have a feel for the natural acoustic of the space they can modify their voice accordingly. Educators would find this equally useful.

Exercises for developing audibility over distance

When using volume to attract attention or issue instructions over distance, the common error is to lock the neck and thrust the head and jaw forwards. The techniques that prove successful in preventing the neck muscles from going into the extreme positions of 'fight or flight/flee' require speakers to inhibit this instinctive reaction, making sure that a free posture and 'grounding' are maintained, and using the imagination to 'draw sound' towards themselves. These exercises work because there is a changed attitude in the speakers who, instead of submitting to the urge to reach out or (in extreme cases) to 'punch' out to the class with their voices, stand their ground and imagine that the voice is beginning at the back of the hall or field and travelling towards them. Sound then flows freely and volume is increased. This will feel very unnatural as first. Repeated exercise is necessary in order to avoid a 'knee-jerk' reaction.

1. **Moving from the wall:** find a spot on the wall and, standing a few inches from it, concentrate on voicing the sound /mah/ and figuratively 'placing' the sound on the spot. Once you have established this placement, keep focusing the sound on the spot but slowly move backwards away from the wall. You may find at first that you run out of breath quite quickly but with practice, this will improve and you will find that you can move further away without loss of breath. It is important to become aware of the sound being drawn away from the point of placement and 'towards' yourself. If this is done successfully, the neck and head never thrust forward and the body remains 'open'. As you continue to do the exercise, increase the arc of sound so that, instead of describing a straight line from the wall to yourself, you allow the sound to arc upwards and over towards you. The arc is used because it explores vocal range, and in speech we use vocal range all the time.

2. **Calling:** imagine that you are on a boat or a mountain top and that you are calling to a friend on another boat or mountain top. Neither point of focus is at an uncomfortable distance but you will need to use an extended sound. Place your hands to your mouth and call in a moderate volume, *Hello there*. The person pretending to be on the second boat or mountain answers, also using the same call. If improvisation is a problem, a simple question and answer such as *How are you?*, *Very well, thank you*, can be planned beforehand. The call is best seen as a continuous sound that lifts and arcs from the mouth of the caller to the ear of the receiver. Shouting should never be used for the exercise, which is about sustaining sound, and it can be done, with practice, with very little volume.

3. **Attracting attention:** use the exclamation *Hey!* in order to attract somebody's attention at the other side of the room. In this exercise it is important to avoid an aggressive approach because in aggressive mode the sound is forced out. The neck and jaw will thrust forward and the habitual laryngeal setting is altered; the larynx is compressed

– often accompanied by vocal discomfort. The fists will often clench, and the shoulder girdle will invariably tighten. The knees will generally lock. It is therefore very important to work in a non-aggressive manner.

Try instead to imagine that the starting point of the sound is from the individual whose attention you want to attract. Instead of pushing the sound out from yourself, draw it towards you. Try using the hands and arms to help you draw the sound slowly over the space until it reaches you. The sound becomes elongated and the vowel /ey/ is used to allow the sound to travel. This helps you to hold your centred physical position. The head need not be thrust forward; in fact you can retain optimum alignment and the neck can remain free, allowing the peripheral vision to be maintained.

4. **Pickpocket exercise:** using the image of drawing sound towards yourself over the space, imagine that you are lifting a scarf out of the pocket of a passer-by. Start by standing fairly close saying the phrase, *The scarf is mine* as you move away from the passer-by. Elongate the vowels and lift and arc the voice, as if it travelled with the scarf from the pocket to you.

   The second part of the exercise is to start further away from the passer-by and vocally 'hook' the scarf and some money out of the imagined pocket. Use the phrase, *The money and scarf are mine.* The use of /m/ aids the voice because it is resonant and a continuous consonant. You should experience a feeling of sustaining sound as you did in the calling exercise.

5. **Fishing exercise:** this is similar to the pickpocket exercise. Imagine a fishing line that you have already cast. Establish where the line and hook have landed and this will become the focal point for your sound. Take in breath easily and without tension; release it on /mah/ as you reel the line in towards yourself. Once the 'drawing towards' of the line has been established, you can develop the exercise by gently increasing volume as the line travels towards you. As with the

other exercises the head and neck should not be thrust forward while voicing.

The principle of all these exercises is that you imagine drawing sound towards yourself rather than pushing it out towards the point of communication. This is quite obviously an image that goes against physical science; nevertheless it keeps the body aligned and is a great aid in the struggle against the tendency to thrust sound out, locking the neck and losing a sense of co-ordinated speech and communication.

Strategies for working over distance and in outdoor spaces

The first involves summoning children when addressing students who may be some distance from you. This, as was discussed above, often leads to the teacher thrusting the head forward and constricting the voice.

- Establish a habit of keeping the group close to you.
- Agree on a 'meeting point' near a wall, tree, or grass bank.
- Ask them to always return to you when an activity is completed and to wait in silence until others have completed their work.
- Use whistles or megaphones to communicate over distance and in so doing avoid the need to shout.

The second strategy is for healthy 'shouting', something which many teachers find vocally challenging.

- 'Call' rather than shout. Calling involves less tension and strain than shouting and achieves better clarity.
- Employ a varied pitch range, even if you feel it is more than you need. Allow vowels to lengthen and become 'musical'. Do not be concerned if you feel you are sounding 'sing-song' as you will eventually find a balance.
- Rather than 'pushing' the voice out of the body, imagine you can 'draw' the sound from where the group is standing towards you.

This change of focus can keep the voice from becoming 'strangulated' or caught in the throat.

The third strategy is simply to increase the audibility of consonants and syllables in order to be clearly understood when addressing a large group.

- Without becoming staccato, losing your rhythm, or diminishing your range, practice enunciating all the consonants in your sentences.
- Pay particular attention to the ends of words.
- Make sure you give syllables their full value. Avoid 'telescoping' or eliding syllables.
- Avoid running one word into another.

Playful exercises for volume

These exercises require a sense of humour because if you feel self-conscious you will hold on to the sound rather than release it. If working with a colleague or fellow staff member, make sure that you both feel that you have created a safe environment in which to work.

1. Using the sound /yah/ /yah/ /yah/ let your jaw be loose and free. Allow yourself to look 'blank or spaced out' and ridiculous.
2. Blow a raspberry /brrr/ or /prrr/ through the lips. This engages and harnesses the breath and you can feel its effects on the lips.
3. Working in pairs, imagine that you are playing tennis. Using an imagined racquet and the sound /doh/ as a ball (any sound beginning with /b/ or /d/ will work), hit the sound very firmly over the 'net' making sure that it reaches your partner. As you get better at sustaining the sound through the air, try lifting and curving the sound. If you are working alone, imagine playing squash.
4. Feel that your weight is centered in the hips and pelvis – imagine that you are dragging yourself through mud. Speak as you do this. 'Three Blind Mice' or any favourite nursery rhyme will do!

5. Sitting on a chair bounce yourself up and down and bounce the sound out as you speak. Try to shake yourself like a 'jelly' while releasing the sounds /ooo/, /aay/, and /ahh/.

6. Lean up against a wall and rhythmically bounce your back against the wall while drunkenly speaking 'Three Blind Mice' – allow the sound to release with each impact.

7. Feel the vibrations in your chest as you sound /mah/. Beat the chest with the fist of one or both hands and allow the sound to release with the impact.

8. Laugh on a low pitch using *ho ho ho*. Do not be concerned if the sound is not genuine. Turn the /ho/ into an elongated call across a distance, lifting and dropping the sound as it travels through the air.

9. Turn the distance call into a phrase such as 'Over here! This way! Ahoy there!' etc.

10. Return to the vowel isolating exercise using the sentence: *How sweet the moonlight sleeps upon this bank!*' (From William Shakespeare, *The Merchant of Venice*, Act V, scene i).

11. In isolation, the vowels are /ow/ /ee/ /u / /oo/ /ai/ /ee/ /u/ /o/ /i/ /a/. Keep 'stringing these vowels together' as if you were speaking the line.

12. Add as much range as you can to the voice as you repeat the vowels. Notice how as you add range and extend the vowels, you also add volume.

13. Repeat the vowels again, laughing as you speak it. Increase the scale of your laughter.

14. Sing the vowels 'operatically' with increased jaw opening and extravagant lip movement.

15. Finally, speak the line as it is written, starting quietly and building volume.

Note: keep the posture aligned at all times.

Volume exercises using verse

White founts falling in the courts of the sun,
And the Soldan of Byzantium is smiling as they run;
There is laughter like the fountains in that face of all men feared,
It stirs the forest darkness, the darkness of his beard,
It curls the blood-red crescent, the crescent of his lips,
For the inmost sea of all the earth is shaken with his ships.

From: G.K. Chesteron, *Lepanto* (circa 1911)

1. Speak the first line on a quiet volume.
2. The next should be louder.
3. The following louder still.
4. Continue until you are as loud as you can be comfortably. Avoid pushing the volume.
5. Keep the neck, head, and shoulders free.
6. Keep the attitude playful and relaxed. Avoid trying too hard.
7. Do not shout or lose support.

When you are happy that you have mastered this exercise, reverse the order, starting loudly and getting quieter.

You can do these exercises walking away and/or towards the wall, increasing volume as you leave the wall and decreasing it as you return to it. Then:

1. Sing a line quietly/speak it quietly with the same support.
2. Sing/speak it with more volume and sustained support.
3. Continue to sing and speak with increasing volume.

Make sure that you add range as you add volume. To explore range, imagine that you are sweeping the voice from the floor to the ceiling. Use all the range at your disposal. Notice how this frees the volume. Then:

1. Count from one to ten getting louder all the time.
2. Repeat the counting exercise very slowly.
3. Repeat once more, making sure that you extend the vowels in each

word. Vowels are voiced and carry both resonance and volume. Do not worry about the strange quality that this produces. The balance between vowel and consonant can be redressed later.

4.   Try speaking a typical classroom phrase, increasing volume each time you speak.

5.   Sing the same phrase, noticing the increased volume, and then speak it once more attempting the same volume.

If the sound is not free, tap the chest or jump up and down to release the sound. Alternatively, sitting on the floor or on a chair bounce, jog or shake the sound out of the body.

It is important to remember that too much effort will block volume rather than create it. Being able to play is an important attribute if volume is the goal.

Although it is important to be able to create volume, it can be a strategy that is over-used. Volume as a norm can be as monotonous as sustained quiet speech. Variety that is responsive and appropriate to the subject matter and situation is ideal. At times it is necessary to look at the alternatives, especially if the voice is suffering.

Trying to produce volume on an ailing voice, whatever the reason, is not advisable.

Volume checklist

The first step is to release the physical tension. A 'checklist' should remind you to:

1.   Release shoulders and neck.

2.   Release jaw and tongue..

3.   Deconstrict the oral space by yawning and smiling.

4.   Open the chest by grasping your hands behind you and stretching arms upwards.

Once this is achieved:

1.   Stand with weight on both feet.
2.   Look at your class or audience and see them as friendly, willing and wanting to hear you. Generally speaking the 'audience', whether learners, students, or strangers, want you to succeed.
3.   Shift the anxiety from yourself and take care of them. That means you want them to have your knowledge or share your experience.
4.   Avoid breath-holding. Breathe out and then allow new air to enter the body just before you begin.
5.   Smile before you start speaking.

This may all seem impossible to begin with but it gets easier as you develop vocal muscle, freedom, and resonance.

Can shouting be healthy?

When asked what is meant by 'shouting' the response is that it is the use of extreme volume and is usually accompanied by emotion, typically anger or frustration. It is the tension that accompanies the emotion that causes the constriction, and can lead to damage.

If increased volume results in a catch in the throat it cannot be healthy. Too often it is a spontaneous emotional response. Professional actors and singers are trained to avoid this tension 'trap' by finding open postures that mimic shouting but that do not lock the breath or the muscles of the throat.

Calmly projected speech and calling is always the best option, but if you find yourself shouting it is important to ensure vocal safety.

It is much more effective to use a controlled and supported sound because any indication of anger suggests a loss of control on the part of the speaker, and this undermines authority, rather than increasing it.

We know that it is possible to use very loud volume without hurting or damaging the voice. Nevertheless many educators can trace a vocal problem back to a specific incident when they, frustrated and angry, have shouted loudly and almost immediately experienced a catch in the throat, a loss of vocal freedom, and a need to force the sound out, resulting in a rough, hoarse, raspy sound with reduced range. They then proceed to attempt to clear the throat but generally to no avail. The loss of control and authority that this can cause is likely to exacerbate any discipline problems that exist.

Children in the playground, however, seem able to shout, call, yell and even shriek with no problems. They are being playful and therefore they are free of negative tension. There is often a quality of laughter lurking beneath the shout which lifts the soft palate and creates space. If you look at their faces you see an open expression that is also mirrored by their posture; the head is aligned, the chest open. The sense of fun removes any tension in the upper body and generally, children are running when they shout and the 'release' that this action gives to the voice avoids the chance of damage. There are exceptions and some children have to be taught to use volume without harming the voice. When competition is introduced even children begin to hurt their voices. Actors are often able to produce blood-curdling cries and yells without damage. It must be said that they have to work at it, to find a technique that works against the emotion of the moment. Creating a 'mock' shout that avoids emotion and sounds authoritative rather than angry can be a useful strategy. It is this technique and a change in emotional response that will allow a loud and commanding use of voice.

All the 'calling' and 'toward' exercises in this section are important for the development of a healthy 'shout', but start with a work-out designed to assist the process; it is important to warm up the voice before attempting the shouting exercises and to precede them with breathing exercises and exercises that release tension in the pharynx and the larynx. If you begin to experience discomfort, it is a signal to stop the exercises and return to breath support work. It is also vital to have a clear idea of your point of focus, i.e., of the individual or groups with whom you wish to communicate. Although the term 'shouting' conjures up ideas of anger, it is never advisable to use high volume if you are angry as it is difficult to separate energy and tension; often, 'inexperienced' shouters are not able to use high energy without constriction, especially if they have to deal with the additional stresses involved in feelings of anger. By removing focus from the larynx and using breath support effectively, a very high volume can be successfully produced without hurting the voice. There are other helpful strategies, such as increasing the precision of the articulation and using a greater than normal vocal range, that remove the need to resort to excessive volume.

There will always be occasions when it is necessary to respond with additional volume and over background noise. It is important to resist an instinctive angry shout response and instead, deliver a supported and healthily executed 'call' or shout. You will be aware by now that in order to produce the clear sound, you need to free the jaw and increase the space in the mouth, use more breath support and 'think' the voice forward and on to the lips. These actions all increase the volume and forward projection of the voice. In addition, lifting the soft palate may help to produce a free clear note when using the voice with volume.

High volume work-out

1. It is important to precede this with work on shoulder, neck and jaw release. It is not recommended that you begin work on shouting until you have developed an awareness of tension that may exist in the jaw and have been able to minimize it. Lift and drop your shoulders 10 times. Turn head from side to side 10 times. Stroke the jaw downwards 10 times. Stretch the tongue as far out of the mouth as you can 10 times, allowing it to return to the mouth slowly. With the tongue tip behind the lower front teeth, bulk the blade of the tongue forward and out of the mouth. Repeat five times feeling the stretch in both the tongue and jaw.

2. Lie on your stomach with a weight on the buttocks and breath down as low in the body as possible. (Your head should be turned to one side and your hands should be shoulder width apart and in line with the ears.) You will feel the buttocks rise as the muscles below the navel move. Develop the exercise by imagining that the breath leaves the body, travelling along each of the vertebrae until it reaches the mouth. Practice this using first the voiceless /fff/ sound and then a gentle hum on /mmm/. Once you have established the journey of the

/mmm/, imagine it begins in the coccyx and increase the energy as it travels up the spine; when you approach the shoulder blades, open the sound into a vowel, e.g. /mmmah/. Repeat the exercise using different vowels such as /mmmaw/ /mmmoh/ /mmmoo/. As you open to the vowel, lift and turn the head to the other side. Allow the voice to change pitch and to lift and arc as you release the sound. As long as you 'begin' the sound well below the level of the larynx, it is possible to develop considerable volume without constriction.

3. The yoga cat: kneel on all fours, and keep your hands directly below the shoulders. As you breathe in, curve the lower back up towards the ceiling as the head tucks in towards the chest. As you breathe out, allow the lower back to sink towards the floor as you imagine the breath moving up through the spine and, as the head comes up and eyes look towards the ceiling, allow the breath to leave the body.

4. After having done this exercise several times on the floor, stand up and vocalize the sustained sound /mmmmmm/ and imagine it travelling up the spine. As it reaches the shoulder blades, open the sound out into /ah/. It may be easier to start in a bent-over position and to unfold through the spine as you produce the sound, synchronizing the movement with the sound.

5. A word of caution: as you release the vowel and lift your eyes upwards do not extend the neck otherwise you may restrict the pharynx.

6. Keep working on this exercise and open to a variety of vowels, e.g. /mmmmmmaw/ /mmmmmmoh/ /mmmmmmay/.

7. Once you are happy with this begin to build volume, feeling the total release of the vowel. Once again never be tempted to start the sound at the level of the larynx. The secret of 'shouting' is to begin the action well below the level of the throat. By picturing the sound starting in the coccyx you remove the focus from the throat. This is of course an image, not a physiological fact, but it helps to keep the sound free. At this stage never get louder than is comfortable and keep the exercises in the style of a call.

8. In pairs, imagine each of you is on the top of a hill, some distance apart. Partner A cups his hands around the mouth and calls to B, *Red roses, who will buy?* B responds, *How much for a dozen?* When this is well established and tension free, use the follow lines:

> A: *Ill met by moonlight, proud Titania!*
> B: *What, jealous Oberon?*

> From: William Shakespeare, *A Midsummer Night's Dream*, Act II, scene i.

9. Repeat the lines again and again, and begin to introduce an attitude of censorship into the dialogue while increasing the volume. Keep monitoring the quality of breath support, space in the mouth and vocal freedom.

10. Now try some of the phrases that you are likely to use in the teaching situation, e.g., *Class four, books away, please, Please hand in your homework*, or *Stand in line please*. Intone the phrase first on one note, then use the hill-calling exercise and thirdly, imagine calling it to the group or child in question.

Further exercises for healthy, high volume voice use

1. Stand back to back with a partner. Bend the knees slightly so that you feel connected, gently and safely supported by each other's weight.

   Using the low breathing muscles around the navel, voice a sustained /hah/and then a /mah/, and visualize the sound travelling through the back (be aware of the resonance in the back). Then begin to introduce phrases such as *Where are you?* The answer from the partner could be *Behind you!* Enjoy the musical rise and fall of the voice and avoid any forcing or striving to achieve quality. Imagine your partner is a long distance from you. Develop this into a 'call' (keeping the body grounded and the head and neck free), then an operatic sound or chant. Finally, imagine you are calling or healthily 'shouting' over background noise. See if you can introduce an element of censorship without creating constriction.

2. Drawing towards (from call to shout): Avoid thrusting the head and neck forward by keeping the body aligned and imagining 'drawing' the voice from a focal point towards yourself. This can be done by imagining attracting someone's attention by summoning them on the 'call' using the sounds /hay!/ or /hi!/. Allow the pitch to rise and fall as the voice travels over distance. Use an arm gesture to 'encourage' the target to approach. Avoid any forward thrust of the jaw, neck and head.

Once an easy open sound has been established, raise the volume. Start quietly and gradually build the volume until projection is achieved. Move into a call and finally a 'shout' over imagined background noise. Avoid constriction in the throat, loss of breath support, and restriction in the oral space.

Monitoring your volume

It is sometimes difficult to judge your own volume, particularly if you speak very loudly or very quietly habitually. Are you louder than you need to be? Sustaining high volume for long periods is tiring for the vocal folds. Monitor your volume when you are not teaching but socializing. Do you use more volume than necessary? Do you attempt to be heard in noisy environments such as pubs and restaurants, in underground stations or crowded rooms?

Remind yourself to use only the necessary volume required and not to chat over loud ambient noise.

Monitor your voice use in the classroom. Ask yourself these questions:

- Do you simply add more noise to the already noisy room?
- Could you use less volume to greater effect?
- Could you speak less?

Chapter outline

- Audibility, volume, projection, clarity, and working in open spaces
- Changing habits
- Common errors
- Adjust your focus
- Posture and Alignment
- 'Grounding' the body and voice
- Exercises to help 'free' the sound from tension
- Creating more sound
- Four quick exercises for creating oral space
- Four quick exercises for forward placement
- The art of projection with pointers from actors
- Consonants plus exercises
- Vowels plus exercises
- Developing resonance
- Varying the pitch
- Exploring volume
- Intention and definition
- Exercises for developing audibility over distance
- Strategies for working over distance and in outdoor spaces
- Playful exercises for volume
- Volume check-list
- Can shouting be healthy?
- High volume work out
- Further exercises for healthy, high volume voice use
- Monitoring your volume

11

More practical work on posture, relaxation, breath, resonance, onset of the note, muscularity, and clarity

Regular work on the voice during the long school holidays and when returning to using the voice professionally after a break can prevent vocal fatigue. This chapter offers further exercises for posture, relaxation, breath, resonance, onset of the note and muscularity for articulation and clarity. The final chapter offers exercises for pitch, vocal variety, and speech-making, and offers warm-up routines.

These exercises can be done by individuals or adapted for different age groups for use in the classroom.

Although for the purposes of addressing specific issues we are separating the different elements of voice production, it is important to remember that the elements are interdependent and should work in harmony. The voice operates best when all its discrete parts work together and support each other.

Posture

When working on your own posture and when addressing postural issues in the classroom remember that work on posture is most effective:

- if weight distribution is equally balanced with feet 15–20 cm (6–8 inches) apart (distribute the weight equally over both feet; imagine that the big toe, little toe and heel form a supportive triangle);

- if the pelvis is balanced and level – avoid thrusting the pelvis too far forward or backward (abdominal muscles should be recruited to help maintain this balance): the pelvis is like a cup filled with tea – tilting it too far forwards or backwards will result in the tea spilling over;
- if a virtual 'space' is maintained between the bottom of the ribcage and the abdominal area by lifting, opening, and relaxing the ribcage while keeping the spine long;
- if the back is expanded sideward and outward, ensuring there is maximum space between the shoulder blades: the back should feel open and broad;
- if shoulders are relaxed and released to their natural level, decreasing tension in the upper chest and shoulder girdle, allowing the arms to hang loosely from the shoulders with the hands and fingers free and relaxed; and
- if the head is poised and balanced on the spinal column so that it can move effortlessly both horizontally and vertically, in order to achieve this, the neck should be free and relaxed – imagine the ears sitting above or 'over' the shoulders, rather than being carried in front of the shoulders in a 'poked forward' manner.

When working on your own posture and when addressing postural issues in the classroom remember that work on posture is of limited effectiveness:

- if posture is over-corrected (quasi-military style) or when spinal alignment loses its easy S shape and becomes rigid and straight;
- if knee joints are locked and thigh muscles are locked and braced resulting in the knees being pushed backward;
- if, when standing, the weight is on one leg only so that one hip juts out, resulting in asymmetry in the area of the pelvis;
- if weight is poorly distributed, for example, if it is too far forward so that the spine is thrown out of alignment resulting in abdominal over-extension;

- if there is constriction in the muscles of the neck, resulting in tension which forces the head back and the chin forward; or
- if high or low eye levels affect the positioning of the head which may lead to tension of the neck muscles.

NB: It takes time to change habitual postures, and new positions may feel uncomfortable initially as new 'muscle patterns' need to be established in order to become familiar and comfortable. The following exercises can also be adapted for use with learners and students. Posture and alignment awareness is particularly beneficial for adolescent classes.

Posture exercises

Work through these exercises yourself before using them with a class.

1. (a) Stand as badly as you can with the weight on one foot, not two, the ribs compressed, the arms folded across the body, the shoulders raised, the head and neck slumped forwards, and the spine curved. Notice how the eye level has fallen.

   (b) Now move from this posture into a more balanced and open position with the weight over both feet; drop the arms to the sides, lengthen the spine, open the rib cage, lower the shoulders, and balance the head on the top of the spine. Notice where the eye level is now. Do not over-correct.

   (c) Repeat this exercise and when you begin to create an open posture, do so by gradually 'internally' adjusting the posture, working through each vertebra individually, 'building' one on top of the other, and gradually sensing that there is greater length to the spine and separation between the hips and floating ribs. Try to 'sense' the muscles releasing and the body realigning. Avoid a sudden external correction.

   (d) Once you are in the balanced position with the knees relaxed and flexible, the pelvis level and not tilted either forwards or backwards, you can begin to stretch. Lift the arms above the head and stretch through the arms to the tips of the fingers while reaching for the ceiling. Look up at the ceiling while you stretch. Keep your heel on the floor and do not lose your balance. The stretch can be maintained for up to 15 seconds before you slowly lower your arms.

2.   As you begin the lowering process, allow the head to lower too. The weight of the head and shoulders will take the spine into a curve, and the movement will eventually involve bending over at the waist and allowing the knees to soften until the body is completely bent over with the arms swinging loosely, touching the floor. Once in this position make sure that the head is free and allowed to hang loosely. The jaw and tongue should be loose and free also. Gradually begin to uncurl by building up one vertebra upon the next until the spine begins to unfold and lengthen. Leave the shoulders, head and neck until last. Once you are completely, but not rigidly upright, repeat the exercise a second and third time.

NB: Moving to an upright position too quickly can occasionally lead to a momentary feeling of dizziness, so uncurl the spine slowly.

3.   Stand with feet slightly apart and weight evenly distributed. The knees should be relaxed, slightly bent but flexible enough to allow them to move back and forward. Check that the pelvis is balanced and the thighs and calves are loose.

4.   Raise the arms above the head but do not extend them to their limit. Interlace fingers quite firmly with the backs of the hands pointing towards the ceiling. Maintain this position but reverse the hands so that, still interlaced, they are now palms upward to the ceiling. Now begin to 'walk' the hands towards the ceiling feeling the lift of the ribcage. Repeat this procedure three or four times. Again notice the space between the lower ribs and the hips.

5.   Stand still with feet slightly apart, and weight evenly distributed, with shoulders relaxed and arms hanging by your sides. The knees should be relaxed, slightly bent but flexible enough to allow them to move back and forward. Check that the pelvis is balanced and the

thighs and calves are loose. Close your eyes and experience the taller, wider and more open posture.

Postural exercise for the classroom

Once the class has established a sense of a free and open body ask the students or learners to work in pairs. One of the pair should create different postures while the partner mirrors them. These postures may include well-aligned positions as well as slumped or over-corrected positions, weight badly distributed on one foot or hip, high shoulders or shoulders that are slumped and rounded, head jutting forward or pulled back. They should aim to finish on an open released posture. This allows the class to feel the difference between positive and negative postures and also to observe the differences.

Shoulders

Most of us hold physical and emotional tension in the shoulders and this can very easily affect the voice because of their proximity to the larynx. Posture is a contributing factor in shoulder tension as is being cold, and carrying heavy bags and equipment. Identifying shoulder tension, and remembering to relax the shoulders regularly throughout the day by shrugging them and re-aligning the head and neck, will make a difference.

Shoulder exercises

Lift the shoulders up to the ears, hold this position for five seconds and then release. Repeat twice more. Then lift the shoulders in a shrug, making sure that they drop fully to a released position. Allow the breath to be released each time the shoulders drop. This should be done several times a day, whenever the shoulders become tense.

1. Lift the shoulders up to the ears, and then move them backwards so that the shoulder blades almost meet. Hold them in this position briefly, before releasing them and moving them forward and upward again. Continue the cycle for at least six rotations.

2. Raise the right arm above the head, stretching through the arm to the fingertips. Notice how the ribcage opens in this position. Take the arm backwards, breathing out as it descends and then complete the circle by lifting the arm up back to the starting point as breath flows back into the body. Repeat this exercise three times on the right side, taking care never to hold the breath but noticing how the opened position of the ribs naturally draws breath in; notice how the downward movement of the ribs expels the air.

3. Repeat the same exercise with the left arm, making sure that you co-ordinate the breath with the action. (Breathe in as the arm is lifted and breathe out as the arm is lowered.)

Neck

When working on your own neck and when addressing neck tension in the classroom remember that work on the neck is most effective:

- if the head is only rotated as far as the shoulders in a relaxed and easy manner;
- if the exercises are undertaken slowly and gently;
- if the eyes lead the movement of the neck; and
- if imagery is used to extend the neck, for example imagine that someone is gently brushing a hand up along the surface of the neck and 'think' the length of the neck rather than physically stretching it.

When working on your own neck and when addressing neck tension in the classroom avoid any work that results in:

- the neck being fully rotated in exercises;
- any discomfort of the neck;
- rigorous movement that places stress on the vertebrae; or
- forced extension of the neck.

Neck exercises

1. Beginning with the head in a balanced position, slowly drop the chin down on to the chest, feeling the extension of the muscles at the back of the neck. Do this three to six times, making sure that no movement is forced. Return the head to a balanced position and feel the length in the back of the neck.

2. Keeping the feeling of length in the back of the neck, but not over-extending it, take the head to the right shoulder and then, keeping the chin close to the chest, move the head slowly to the left shoulder. Repeat, starting at the left shoulder and moving towards the right one. Never rotate the head fully or do any neck exercises hurriedly.

3. Keeping the head balanced on the top of the spine, alternately lift and sway each shoulder up and down in a 'wave-like' motion. Keep the movement fluid and relaxed.

4. Using the image of the head balanced on a greasy ball-bearing at the top of the spine, allow the head to bob gently using gentle movements rather like those of a marionette.

Relaxation

When working on your own relaxation and when addressing relaxation issues in the classroom remember that work on relaxation is most effective:

- when relaxation exercises are conducted in a space that is warm, comfortable, and conducive to relaxation;
- if clear explanations of relaxation techniques are given and understood so as to maximize the possibility of successful execution of exercises;
- when the pitch, speed, and volume with which instructions are given are monitored in order to create an environment conducive to relaxation;
- when age-appropriate exercises for individuals and groups are selected in order to maximize the likelihood of success;

- when exercises used for relaxation are varied and incorporate differ-ent positions such as lying, sitting, standing, and moving about;
- when participants can identify habitually held areas of tension through kinesthetic and body awareness;
- when using imagery to work on relaxation – individuals should be encouraged to select personal images that are restful and relaxing;
- when participants develop awareness of the difference between ten-sion and relaxation;
- when good alignment is encouraged, because a slumped position is rarely a relaxed position; and
- when you allow yourself or students enough time to emerge from a deeply relaxed state.

When working on your own relaxation and when addressing relaxa-tion issues in the classroom remember that work on relaxation is of limited effectiveness:

- without comprehension and application of the principles behind relaxation and their role in vocal effectiveness;
- without developing the ability to distinguish between states of ten-sion and release;
- when exercises are delivered quickle and with tense vocal quality;
- in stressful situations and with demanding and stress-inducing workloads;
- when working on relaxation in physically cramped, cold, or uncom-fortable conditions;
- when insufficient time is allocated for exercises; or
- when insufficient time is given to emerge from the deeply relaxed state.

Relaxation exercises

There are two very effective methods of relaxing on your own. The first is through a 'stretch and release' method and the second is through the use of image and the establishment of a feeling of release in the muscles that you are able to isolate. Relaxation through imagery can be carried out independently and suits many individuals. It may require time to establish the 'feeling' of relaxation but once this is achieved, it is possible to self-monitor progress effectively.

For most people, the tensions that they carry become habitual and are therefore difficult to isolate and to identify in specific muscles. Working to identify tension is the first step towards releasing it. When working with a class, a combination of approaches would be wise in order to appeal to students with different learning preferences. The following exercises can be adapted to any age:

Stretching

1. Kneel on the floor, sit back on your heels, and stretch the arms forward along the floor so that you feel the stretch in the spine. Hold the stretch for a few seconds and then release it.

2. Lie on your back on the floor with arms and legs in a star shape. Now stretch diagonally so that the right arm and left leg are stretched away from the centre of the body. Hold then release. Then stretch the left arm and the right leg. Hold then release. Feel the sense of breadth in the back.

3. You can do the following exercise either sitting in a chair or lying on the floor. If in a chair make sure that you are comfortable with sufficient support for your neck and lower back. If lying on the floor you may want to place a book under your head and bend your legs at the knee in order to reduce the curve in the lower back. In this exercise you issue instructions to yourself, beginning with the command to 'create and hold tension', then to release it and finally, to assess the new muscle state. The aim of the exercise is to teach the body to differentiate between habitually held tension and the released state.

    (a) Starting with the head, push it into the floor, the book or the back of the chair. Hold the tension. Release the tension and then assess the different sensations in the muscles of the neck and those around them.

(b)   Now push the shoulder girdle into the back of the chair or the floor. Give the self-instructed command 'hold'. After a few seconds self-instruct to 'release'. Then 'assess' the difference between the states of tension and release.

(c)   Move on to the back. Push the spine into the floor or into the back of the chair. Hold the tension and then release and assess. Continue through the body, tightening and releasing buttocks, arms, fists, legs, feet, jaw, and finally, the whole body.

Once you begin to identify and isolate tension successfully, you can create and hold tension on the left side of the body while leaving the right side released and vice versa. This can be extended to holding tension in the right leg and left arm while the opposite limbs are relaxed. When isolating to this extent it is important to keep monitoring the neck and keeping it free.

Image relaxation

Once more, get comfortable either on a chair or on the floor. Make sure that you are warm. Think of a place you would like to be; imagine somewhere tranquil such as on a warm beach, in a field of flowers or on a gently rocking boat on a calm, blue sea.

Use the image to create a feeling of peace. Imagine the feeling of the sun on your limbs. If possible play some relaxing music. Concentrate on the feeling that in this ideal setting you have no responsibilities or worries. Try to recreate the experience of being on holiday.

Now work through the body from the feet upwards, ensuring that each part of the body is relaxed. If you are not happy with the state of tension in a group of muscles, tighten the muscles in question and then release them. Work up slowly through the legs, pelvis and buttocks, spine, ribcage, chest, shoulders and arms, hands, fingers, neck, head, and facial muscles.

Breathing

When working on your own breathing and when addressing breathing issues in the classroom remember that work on breath is most effective:

- when a clear, concise explanation of the anatomy and physiology of breathing is given;
- if breathing exercises are practiced when the body is in a relaxed state;
- if a well aligned posture is maintained in order to encourage an open ribcage and maximize rib swing;
- if particular attention is paid to establishing a relaxed open shoulder position that is not rounded or hunched;
- if the ribs are released and exercised before breathing exercises begin;
- if the degree of upper chest movement is limited by ensuring that the shoulders are relaxed and the lower muscles used in breathing are engaged;
- if a routine of relaxed, aligned, and effortless breathing is established, ensuring optimum lung capacity;
- when participants understand the significance of inspiration and expiration, and the way in which breath supports voice and aids effective communication;
- if stretching and relaxation of the back to maximize lung expansion is part of the exercise routine;
- when practice in the control of the breath cycle is undertaken regularly;
- when scenarios in which different amounts of air for voicing in specific situations such as singing, speaking quietly, calling, etc. are explored;
- when breathing is easy and silent, indicating relaxed, open airways and a body that is poised but not stressed;
- when attention is paid to the lower back and the abdominal muscles which play an important part in the breathing process: it is impor-

tant that the muscles in these areas are not locked and can therefore support the easy movement of muscles involved in healthy breathing;

- when the phrase 'breathe down/breathe wide' is used rather than the phrase 'take a big breath' which can create tension; and
- if the focus is on breathing out, the subsequent in-breath will occur much more naturally.

When working on your own breathing and when addressing breathing issues in the classroom remember that work on breath is of limited effectiveness:

- if too much focus is on the breathing-in phase as it can lead to tension in the upper chest and hyper-ventilation;
- if too much effort causes movement in the shoulders and neck in an attempt to create a full breath;
- if participants lack awareness of the amount of air needed for voice as insufficient breath leads to breathy, unstable delivery;
- if there is an inability to manage the outgoing breath stream, resulting in letting breath out in a rush at the beginning of a phrase or sentence;
- when breath-holding and speaking on too little breath at the beginning of the phrase or sentence results in the breath being released too late to be used effectively;
- if excessively rapid breathing cycles (over-breathing) lead to hyperventilation, causing a feeling of light-headedness as a result of too much oxygen being absorbed into the bloodstream too quickly;
- when working on breathing exercises with poorly aligned posture: it should be neither over-corrected nor slumped; or
- when the body holds excessive tension: tension is spread quickly throughout the body and manifested in the upper body and vocal tract, resulting in a noisy intake of breath.

Rib exercises

It is important to work on opening the ribs as preparation for work on the breath.

1. Raise the right arm above the head, stretching it towards the ceiling. Slowly rotate the arm in a circular movement, first backwards and then forwards, watching it as it moves back upwards. Repeat five backward circles followed by five forward circles.

2. Standing with the right foot forward and the right knee slightly bent, lean your weight forward from the waist, curving the back as you bring the arms over the knee. Keep the elbows slightly bent and the hands in a soft fist just above the knee. Allow the spine to curve forward and the torso and ribs to become concave. The hands should 'hover' just above the knee.

3. Then sweep the arms backwards and out to your sides as far as is comfortable as you shift your weight onto your back (left) leg. The arms should be open in this position and held at shoulder height with the palms of the hands facing upwards. The front leg should straighten as the back knee bends and supports the weight. Notice how, as you lean backwards and open the body, the ribcage widens and opens and breath enters the lungs.

4. Reverse the action by bending forward and returning the arms to the knee, noticing as you do that the ribs close in and breath leaves the body as the spine curves forward.

5. Repeat this exercise five times and then change feet so that the left foot is forward and the right foot is behind. Start with the weight on the left foot and the knee slightly bent. Repeat the exercise five times on this side.

6. Begin standing with the arms by your sides hanging loosely from the shoulders. Grasp a 'stretchy exercise band' with both hands, about 15 cm/6 inches apart (use the more flexible coloured bands: yellow,

red, or green). The starting position is with the shoulders and arms relaxed and hands alongside the thighs.

7.   Slowly lift the band above the head.

8.   Stretch the band to enable you to take it over the head so that it moves to behind your back. Notice how the ribcage is opened in this movement.

9.   Slowly return the band over your head and down to the knees.

10. Repeat five times.

This exercise can also be done in a sitting position.

NB: Do not do this exercise if it hurts or if you have an existing shoulder problem or injury.

Breathing exercises

1.   Lie on the floor in a comfortable position with a small book under your head and with your legs bent at the knee to reduce the curve in the lower back. Relax the shoulder girdle. Place a book, or better still a small brick, below the ribcage or just below the waistline. Relax either by doing one of the exercises in the relaxation section above, or by simply resting for a few minutes. Notice how, as you begin to relax and breathe, the action of the diaphragm gently pushes the book or brick upwards as breath enters the body and begins to fall as breath leaves the body.

2.   Relax the shoulders so they are not involved in the breathing process. As you breathe out allow the air to leave the body on a gentle /fff/. Once the air has left the body, wait for the body to 'need' a new breath before taking one; if you over-breathe you will feel dizzy. It is important to breathe out at a slower speed than you breathe in. Notice how a rhythm develops. The breath comes in to an internal count of three or four; there is a slight pause and then the breath leaves to a count of four or five. There should also be a pause before the new breath is inhaled.

3.   Lying on your stomach, get your head into a comfortable position; most people find lying with the face to one side is best. Place a heavy book or brick on to the buttocks so that you can feel it rise and fall as you breathe in and out. This is a useful exercise because it allows you to feel the breath in a way that is impossible when you stand up; as you are lying on the abdomen, the action of the diaphragm when breathing in results in displacement of the internal abdominal organs. You are able to feel this as movement in the lower back and buttocks. It is also good for creating a feeling of 'separation' in the lower vertebrae, and allowing relaxation in muscles in an area in which many of us hold tension.

4.   Standing in front of a mirror, place one hand on the midriff. As you breathe out, place some pressure on the midriff and notice how the outgoing breath results in the muscles below the hand moving towards the spine. As breath comes into the body the hand will follow the muscles of the midriff outwards. While you are doing this, check in the mirror that the shoulders are not lifting significantly as breath comes in. Begin to develop a more conscious outward breath using /fff/ to the count of five. Pause, and then feel the breath come in under the hand to the count of three, followed by /fff/ out again to the count of five. Once confident with these exercises, increase the duration of the outgoing breath from five to seven or eight. Never force this; what is important is that you become conscious of the fact that the ribcage and abdomen expands as breath comes in and decreases in size as breath is exhaled.

5.   Stand with your hands stretched outwards in a star position. Breathe out on /s/ and as you do so bend over to touch the floor, allowing your knees to bend as you go over. Pause until you feel the need to breathe. When the need is felt, stand up and return to your original position and feel the breath re-entering the body as space is created. The object of this exercise is to illustrate that the open body position

produces an effortless intake of breath and, when the ribcage is not constricted, breath freely enters the body.

Are you a breath-holder?

For some teachers the problem is associated more with learning to release breath than with learning to breathe in. We often stop ourselves breathing out fully, either consciously or unconsciously, through tension and subsequently create a shallow in-breath.

The fight-or-flight/flee response has been examined in **Chapter 4**. When we feel excitement, anticipation, fear, or are under stress of any sort, a common reaction is to lock the neck and shoulders and hold the breath. Many teachers are familiar with the physical feeling of being 'locked' that results from a degree of panic. When we hold breath or 'fix' the head and neck, we immediately become 'bound' and lose our ability to be responsive to the world around us. We are usually very aware of the need to take breath in, in order to prepare for speech, but often do not release the breath as we speak, resulting in a sound that is not breath supported. The advice to 'breathe out' when under pressure may seem very simplistic but it is very helpful. With the outgoing breath, many held tensions are released.

Exercises for releasing held breath

Here are some exercises that will help you to stop 'holding and fixing'.

1. Using a voiceless sound, such as /ff/, /ss/, /sh/, or /th/, feel the breath pass over the tongue or lips as it is released.
2. Raise and drop the shoulders, releasing the breath as you let the shoulders fall.
3. Sigh out deliberately and noisily, expelling breath not voice.
4. Stretch up to the ceiling and then collapse from the waist, releasing the breath as you do so.
5. Imagine that you need to push a car up a hill. As you prepare for the action the breath fills the lungs; as you 'push' you will notice that you contain the breath within the lungs (the ribcage remains open.)

Once you have completed the action and reached your goal and you relax, you will notice how the surplus breath leaves the lungs. Repeat several times noticing the preparation, holding and release of the breath.

6. Standing with feet wide apart stretch arms out to the side and lengthen the spine and neck, making the body as broad and as long as possible. Hold the position for a few seconds and then release the arms. Notice that the breath, which has been held, is also released. Avoid 'slumping' and shortening the spine.

7. Now repeat the previous body position and this time, make sure that you do not hold the breath but instead, actively free the neck and abdominal muscles and breathe in and out freely while keeping the spine long.

8. Imagine that you are eager to speak but as soon as you are about to begin someone else speaks first. Notice the momentary holding of breath each time you are interrupted.

9. Imagine that you are blowing the seeds off a dandelion. To begin with use a long sustained breath. Then try blowing five short sharp blasts of breath to remove all the seeds. Make sure that your breath action comes from the centre of the body.

10. Imagine that you are bouncing a ball using one hand. As you bounce the ball release the breath on /pah/. Then experiment by holding your hand to your mouth and feel the breath on your hand.

11. Using your arm as a scythe, engage the breath to produce the sound /fff/ as you 'slice through long grass'. Begin with one 'slice' on one breath and build to four separate 'slices' on one breath.

12. Imagine that you are performing a martial art and 'punch and slice' the air releasing breath as you do so. Explore different qualities of breath on /fff/, /sh/, /sss/, /ttt/, /ppp/, and /kkk/ as you move. Use the consonants only and do not add a vowel as this will introduce voice.

13. Using an imaginary ball, roll it across the floor on a smooth sound-less stream of breath. 'Follow' it to its destination with both the arm

and the breath. Repeat using /fff/, /sss/ and then introduce voice on /mah/, /moo/, and /maw/.

14. Holding your hand up to your mouth release a thin stream of breath on to your hand silently. Then with a wide-open throat, breathe all your breath out silently through a relaxed, open throat and mouth on to your hand. You should feel the broad column of warm air but hear no sound at all. If you hear a rasping noise, there is tension in the throat. Make sure that you 'feed' the breath through from the low abdominal muscles.

Having done these exercises you should have experienced what it feels like to hold on to breath and release it. Once you can identify the sensation, you are well on the way to learning to release it. Try to catch yourself holding your breath. If you do, make sure that you release your shoulders, neck and jaw and actively breathe out. If the occipital joint at the base of the skull and the top of the spine is locked, free exchange of breath is unlikely so it is important to work on neck exercises in order to free this point.

Resonance

Resonance is a complex phenomenon which depends on multiple vocal criteria. In order to promote balanced resonance, aspects pertaining to resonance will be addressed in the exercises.

When working on your own resonance and when addressing resonance issues in the classroom, remember that work on resonance is most effective:

- if there is regular use of exercises to establish a relaxed and free vocal tract;
- if the jaw, tongue, cheeks, and lips have been exercised and negative tension has been released;
- if a kinesthetic awareness of the resonators through work on vibrations has been explored;
- if practical and playful auditory training has been undertaken through games and mimicry;

- if an understanding of the importance of the oral resonators and the lips and tongue in the formation of vowel sounds exists, and the relationship between resonators and accent has been established;
- if an awareness of any imbalance in the resonators has been acknowledged;
- if a full explanation of any possible medical reasons for an imbalance of resonance is given and understood;
- when awareness of different resonance within particular cultural, ethnic or language groups has been encouraged;
- when other cultural resonance is explored as a way to free up habitual use of resonance and offer alternatives; and
- if there is an understanding of the physical relationship between the resonators: how tension contributes to and restricts vibration, and how individuals can choose to alter the balance of resonance.

When working on your own resonance and when addressing resonance issues in the classroom remember that work on resonance is of limited effectiveness:

- if working on resonance before releasing, relaxing, and aligning the whole body;
- if working on resonance without paying specific attention to the release of tension in the vocal tract, the muscles of the jaw, the lips and cheeks, the mask of the face, and the root of the tongue;
- if working on specific resonators before doing exercises to ensure the head, throat and neck are fully released, mobile, and relaxed;
- if working on resonance without a clear understanding of the way in which the size, shape, and texture of the resonating cavity affects the fundamental note, and how changes can be made to vocal quality by altering the shape, size, and texture of resonators;
- if working without an understanding of the way in which resonators are connected and how different resonators affect the vocal quality;

- if working without an appreciation of harmonics and the way that the natural harmonies of the voice are reinforced by finding sympathetic shapes and textures within the resonating cavities;
- if there is a lack of awareness of the resonators and their role in developing resonance;
- without the knowledge of the ways in which resonance is transferred to other resonators;
- if there is a lack of auditory training; or
- if chronic medical issues such as nasal congestion, allergies, and adenoids have not been treated.

Resonance exercises

We recommend the following exercises are done in preparation for work on resonance:

1. Keep the lips together with light contact and then try to produce a full yawn or even an attempted or half-yawn.

2. Try to imagine chewing gum or toffee which increases in size with every chewing movement. As you do this you will be aware of the increased size and openness of the pharynx.

3. Try an 'inside' smile. In this exercise you relax the lips and 'smile' with the back of the mouth in the area of the oropharynx or where you feel the tonsils might be. The inside smile will increase your awareness of this area and encourage you to open it up. Some people find it easier to think of being an opera singer attempting to hit a very high note. Take up the posture of the effort but do not make any sound. This will give a sense of the placement of the inside smile.

4. Deliberately create tension in the jaw, tongue, and pharynx and speak a sentence in a very tight nasal way. It is useful to contrast the sound and sensation that you have when speaking in this manner with the sound and sensation that you have when the sentence is spoken without tension.

5. Repeat and contrast the full mellow sound that you achieve with an open relaxed pharynx with that of a tight constricted pharynx which results in a harsh metallic sound.

6. Speak the line *Here we go round the mulberry bush* with a very loose jaw as if you were slightly drunk, and then again as if your teeth were stuck together *Owen ought to go to Orlando.*

7. The purpose of this next exercise is to explore the potential of the resonance and pitch of the voice beyond that used habitually. For introverts it can be daunting, but it can also be a lot of fun. Imagine you are providing the voice for a cartoon character.

   Using the rhyme 'Three blind mice' create a 'voice' you associate with the following animals: a snake, a bear, an elephant, a giraffe, a canary, a St Bernard dog, a cat, a cow, a parrot, an ape, a moose, and a lion. Finding the physicality of the animal can help create an alternative sound. Do not worry about stereotyping the animal sound at this point.

Exercises for oral resonance

Before starting work on oral resonance, make sure the mouth is open and relaxed by yawning, and release the tongue by stretching it outside the mouth and gently stroking the jaw downwards to release the temporomandibular joint around the jaw 'hinge'.

1. An easy exercise is to start from a yawn and move into a sigh. Monitor the different sound produced in relation to the degree of oral space, first with a limited space and then with a free, open oral space.

2. Speak the line *The five parked cars are mine* with a tight jaw, tense tongue, and restricted oral space. Then repeat with a loose jaw, relaxed tongue, and open oral space.

3. You can try the same combination of movements with these sentences:

Now I see the fleecy clouds.
Not hot rolled gold, but cold rolled gold.
Mark Parker sent a letter to settle the bet.

4. As further practice, the following sentences may be used, focusing on giving the vowels their full value:

The five parked cars are mine
> (vowels /ai/ as in *high* and /ah/ as in *park*)

Now I see the fleecy clouds
> (/ee/ as in *see* and /ow/ as in *now*)

Cold and hot rolls are sold a lot
> (/oh/ as in *cold* and /o/ as in *hot*)

Owen ought to go to Portsmouth in the morning
> (/aw/ as in *Paul* and /oh/ as in *cold*)

5. In order to experience the difference that lip shape and oral space make to a vowel's pitch and resonance, use the sound /woo/ to mimic the sound of the wind, play with lip shape and cadence.

6. Using breath only, breathe through the following vowels below and listen to the pitch produced when the vowel is shaped loosely (maintaining optimum space) and when it is shaped tightly (reducing space).

/oo/ as in *cool*
/u/ as in *would*
/oh/ as in *cold*
/aw/ as in *Paul*
/o/ as in *hot*
/ah/ as in *park*
/u/ as in *hut*
/er/ as in *curl*
/e/ as in *set*
/ay/ as in *make*

/i/ as in *it*

/ee/ as in *sea*

Try speaking the same vowels with tighter or looser lip positions. Listen to the change in quality that this gives to the vowels.

7.   Try the same exercise, but this time with a higher or lower tongue position. Return to the shape that feels most effective. Remember the position and try to use it again.

It is important to note that different regional accents will produce different resonant pitch.

Exercises for pharyngeal resonance

The pharyngeal resonator is closely aligned to the oral and nasal resonators through the oropharyngeal and nasopharyngeal openings into the pharynx. It is a mobile and readily altered space. The pharynx is sensitive to changes in posture, tension and muscle configuration, and is responsive to emotional stress. Exercises to develop increased pharyngeal resonance are very useful, not only in enhancing the resonance of the voice by finding a connection with the chest but also, in releasing areas of tension in the jaw and tongue.

1.   Create an open and released oral cavity by moving into a yawn, feeling the increase in size of the oropharynx with a corresponding increase in the distance between the upper and lower molars. In this exercise it is most important to concentrate on the increased space at the back rather than the front of the mouth. Too much space at the front of the mouth will lead to tension in the area of the jaw 'hinge' (temporomandibular joint).

2.   Relax the jaw and allow a limited opening at the front of the mouth. Produce an 'inside smile' at the back of the oral cavity. This might bring on a yawn; if so, allow it to develop and feel the expansion of the pharynx.

3.   Let the tongue protrude as much as is comfortably possible and attempt to speak a sentence clearly. It is the effort to achieve clarity

that will open up the pharyngeal space. Obviously the sound will not be natural, but that is not a requirement of this exercise. Relax and feel the space created. Monitor the effect by repeating the same sentence without protruding the tongue. Added resonance should have been achieved.

4.   From a yawn move into a sigh as you breathe out. Use /ah/ or /aw/ for practice because this will encourage space in the mouth as well as in the pharynx. Your tongue tip should be touching the lower front teeth but should not be pressed against them.

5.   Once you have established the yawn, sigh out on /oh/ and then say the following sentences keeping the pharynx as relaxed as possible.

'I'd only own a golden opal', said Owen.
Over and over and over again Mo told that old story.
Only Omar owns a gold Roller.
Only old soldiers own those overcoats.

6.   Establish a yawn and then from the yawn move into a sigh on the out breath. The vowel /ah/ or /aw/ is recommended as this will encourage maximum oral and pharyngeal space. The tongue should be relaxed with the tip in contact with the lower front teeth.

The car would not start as a sparkplug was worn.
Farmer Martin farms calves in Dartmouth.
Audrey and Aubrey almost always order four portions.
Paul saw the larks soar at dawn.

7.   Contrast the vocal tone of the open, relaxed pharynx with a tight constricted pharynx, which gives a harsh metallic sound, by breathing through the sound /hah/ initially with an open and relaxed pharynx, with the tongue relaxed and flat in the mouth and tongue tip touching the lower front teeth.

Contrast this with the same sound /hah/ made with a tight pharynx, tight bunched tongue and reduced jaw opening.

8. Using the sentence *Eve ate apples all afternoon*, listen to the sound achieved when contrasting:

- excessively loose cheek muscles with excessively tight cheek muscles;
- a raised soft palate with a lowered soft palate;
- a retracted tongue with a forward, floppy tongue; and
- clenched teeth with an excessively open jaw.

Exercises for nasal resonance

The nasal resonators are the least adaptable in terms of their ability to change shape and size, but they are of considerable significance in the effect they have on voice quality. Extremes of disordered nasal resonance may occur as a consequence of certain oral and maxillofacial disease or inappropriate vocal placement held in the area of the oropharynx. Some regional accents make greater use of nasal resonance than others, and it is generally accepted that American English is more nasally resonated than British English. Tension in the soft palate and tongue can produce a tight nasal sound. It is important when working on nasal resonance to achieve a balance between oral, pharyngeal, and nasal resonators.

1. The /ng/ sound as in *song* and *ring*, and the /m/ and /n/ sounds lower the soft palate and will produce nasal resonance. Produce the following sounds in sequence:

/ng ah/ng oh/ng ee/
/n ah/n oh/n ee/
/m ah/m oh/m ee/

Make sure that the contrast between the nasal consonant and the denasalized vowel is established initially by separating the sounds and subsequently moving to a blend. Repeat the exercise five times.

2. The following sentences are useful practice material for developing nasal resonance. Once again maintain the contrast between nasal consonants /m/n/ng/ and the non-nasal vowel.

Martha's marvellous mother makes mouthwatering mousaka.

Noel is missing singing songs in Singapore.

Ryan enjoys ringing bells in Tonga.

Calling Nancy nasty names is never nice.

Never knowingly munch on mackerel nocturnally.

It never snows in Nigeria, Namibia, or Nicaragua in the winter months.

Marleen Mary Methuan may buy some mangoes from the market in Mandalay.

Many morose men make much money on Mondays.

Many melancholy milk maids miserably moan about the noisy nanny goats.

November is not the month for munching many mince pies.

Nora the nice nurse never nurses noisy naughty children.

In Nottingham nine hundred and ninety-nine nesting nightingales noisily sing and dance in the nearly night sky.

The morbid musicians mournfully murmur the mystical madrigal.

Norman's nautical submarine was knocked by the naughty ninja from Nan Tong.

My mice make magnificent mountains from many nibbled cushions.

Such nonsensical sentences are nothing but a nuisance to the innocent onlooker.

There is room for improvisation here and students can help by making up sentences as well. Working on the nasal resonators is more difficult because there is less 'room for manoeuvre'. Some teachers will speak with regional accents that make greater or lesser use of nasal resonance. The reason for working on nasal resonance is to achieve a balance of oral, nasal, and pharyngeal resonance.

Exercises for chest resonance

1. Sounding a sustained /m/ and opening to the vowel /ah/, gently beat the chest with both fists. Repeat the exercise using /v/ and opening to the vowels /oh/, /aw/, and /oo/.

2. Using the sound /vah/ or /mah/ or /zah/, move from a note in the middle of the range, gliding down into the chest register, decreasing in intensity and monitoring the sound very carefully to avoid a 'pushed' feeling. It is particularly important that young women should not strive to push the voice down thinking that this will give them more authority.

3. Standing with a well aligned posture, place the hands on the bony structure of the upper chest. Feel the resonance while singing or chanting a descending scale of four or five notes on all the following sustained sounds:

/m/
/v/
/z/
/zh/

Start at different points in the range, exploring the resonance and pitch.

4. Repeat the exercise, opening onto the vowel /ah/, then /oh/, then /aw/. Do not push the voice below a comfortable note, but try to experience chest resonance and feel the vibration of the sound in the front and back of the body.

5. For professional voice users it is important to identify the dominant resonator and to develop the under-used resonators. Of particular importance for actors is the ability to switch selectively from one resonator to another for character work; this can be a useful skill for teachers who read to classes.

6. Without forcing or straining the voice, speak the following sentences, selecting which resonator to prioritize: either the chest, oral space, pharynx, mask of the face, or head. Keep this exercise playful:

    My money may go missing.
    Vivienne vies for violets.
    Zoe is a zebra at the zoo.

7. Beat the chest with the fists while exploring the vowels in this poem:

    There is sweet music here that softer falls
    Than petals from blown roses on the grass,
    Or night-dews on still waters between walls
    Of shadowy granite, in a gleaming pass;
    Music that gentlier on the spirit lies,
    Than tir'd eyelids upon tir'd eyes …

    From: Alfred Tennyson, *The Lotos-Eaters*

Forward placement

Forward placement aids balanced resonance and it is therefore suggested that the following exercises form part of a resonance 'work out'.

Exercises for forward placement

1. Using the sound /yee/ (as in yield), create a megaphone shape with the mouth and lips, and place the hands on the forehead; feel the vibrations. Experiment with pitch in order to explore the vibration.

2. Place the fingers over the nose to block it and speak the following sentence.

    This is the house that Jack built.

    If there is any nasal 'popping' or nasal sound, the voice is not forward enough on the lips.

3. Using the same sentence, with fingers over the nose, work in an 'incorrect' way and create a nasal sound in order to identify the dif-

ference between forward and backward placement. Notice how adding greater breath support, releasing the jaw and creating more space in the oropharynx allows the resonance to shift forward.

4.   Begin with a tight nasal tone and gradually bring the voice forward and 'out of the nose'. Once you have identified the kinesthetic experience of forward placement, remove the fingers from over the nose and repeat the sentence with forward placement.

Healthy voicing: de-constriction and onset of the note

In an effort to avoid damage to the vocal folds when moving from silence into voice it is important to bring the vocal folds together smoothly and gradually as the sound is produced. This avoids the vocal folds coming together with too much tension, which causes them to make an abrupt and tight contact. This closure interrupts the airstream for an instant and the air is released explosively. The sound produced is heard as a hard or glottal 'attack' at the onset of voicing, and it is particularly noticeable when words begin with a vowel when the speaker is stressed.

When working on your own onset and when addressing onset issues in the classroom remember that work on onset is most effective:

- with a relaxed and open attitude to the exercises;
- when shoulders, neck, jaw, and tongue are relaxed and free;
- when the onset of the note is accompanied by a relaxed physicality and open jaw position;
- if breath is adequate and well controlled in order to support the voice; and
- with good co-ordination between the muscles of breathing and the muscles of voice.

When working on your own onset and when addressing onset issues in the classroom remember that work on onset is of limited effectiveness:

- if undue laryngeal tension is present as it will compromise the movement of the vocal folds and may result in a harsh breathy note;
- if excessive pharyngeal tension exists as it may give rise to a feeling of general tension/tightness in the neck;
- if there is upper chest and shoulder tension present which may result in a pushed and strident vocal quality;
- if there is limited control over the in-breath which will reduce the volume of air breathed in and thus affect the amount of breath support available for the voice;
- if the voice is produced on the in-breath; or
- when the outgoing breath is not synchronized with the onset, causing a glottal onset of the note.

Before attempting onset exercises it is important to eliminate constriction in the area of the jaw, oropharynx, pharynx, and larynx as this results in harsh onset and diminished and/or misplaced resonance.

Constriction is usually the result of:

- a clenched jaw and teeth;
- tension in the root of the tongue (with the tongue pushing against the upper palate or bunched and drawn back in the mouth); or
- neck and shoulder tension.

De-constriction exercises

Before working on onset exercises it is important to remove constriction from the vocal area. To release the jaw joint (hinge), gently stroke the jaw down slowly to create space between molars at the back of the mouth.

1. Exercise the jaw hinge/joint by sliding it forward so that the lower front teeth are pushed forward of the upper front teeth. Repeat the action several times moving the lower jaw in a downward circle. Repeat several times. The gentle stretch should be felt in the muscles of the jaw hinge. Never over-extend the joint.

2. With the tongue tip tucked behind the lower front teeth, slowly bulge the body of the tongue forward and out of the mouth – feel the stretch in the jaw and tongue.

3. Raise awareness of your inner pharyngeal posture by first yawning and then feeling the sense of space between the upper and lower molars by lifting the soft palate in an expression of surprise, or opening the eyes wide and imitating an opera singer's facial posture.

4. The yoga lion: suddenly (and simultaneously) stretch fingers with eyes widely open while stretching the tongue out of the mouth. Hold the position briefly and then gently release; the eyes, jaw, and tongue will slowly return to their natural positions where they remain relaxed and neutral. Experience and savour the space inside the mouth and oropharynx.

5. Place an imaginary seed on the back of the tongue. Imagine it is planted and begins to sprout. As it does so, accommodate the growth by adjusting the space in the area of the jaw hinge/joint and the oropharynx.

6. Holding an imaginary glass or large mug, tip the contents slowly over the back of the tongue and down the oesophagus – feel the additional space that has been created.

7. Stretch the tongue out of the mouth – release it and leave it touching the lower front teeth, then try to speak as clearly as possible.

8. While placing one hand on the breathing muscles in the centre of the body, breathe out silently onto an imaginary mirror held in the other hand as if you were 'misting it up'. Be aware of the direct connection between the breath you initiate in the low breathing muscles and the warmth you feel on your hand. Make certain that the breath both enters and leaves the body silently and without tension.

When you have achieved this, add a gentle 'touch of sound' such as a pleasurable /aah/ or /ooh/ sigh.

Onset exercises

When producing an /h/ sound the vocal folds do not fully approximate, which limits the likelihood of the vocal folds 'banging' together to produce a hard glottal attack. Exercising onset by producing an /h/ sound can develop auditory and kinesthetic awareness and enable identification of the difference between smooth onset and hard attack.

It is important to be aware that the /h/ sound should be produced as a gentle /huh/, rather like the sound heard when breathing out as though in annoyance. The sound should be easy, not forced.

1. Create an 'inside smile' as if you were smiling with the muscles in the back of the mouth in the area of the molars and uvula. You should feel as if you are about to initiate a yawn. You will become aware of the space at the back of your tongue and your lifted soft palate. Creating this space is very helpful when working on the onset of the note, volume, and 'healthy shouting'.

2. First, breathe in and then out silently. Then breathe in and out on /h/. Repeat several cycles of both the silent and /h/ breath. Add /ah/ to the /h/ sound so that the sound /hah/ is heard. Repeat this several times keeping the sound relaxed. Listen to the sound carefully, noting any tension in the voice.

3. Repeat this exercise but use different vowels such as /aw/, /oh/, and /uh/. Try to avoid the use of /ee/ as this can sometimes cause undue tongue and lip tension. Try the following:

   /hey/ /hoh/ /huh/ /hai/ /hoo/ /hah/

4. Then drop the /h/ and speak the vowel with a gentle onset while maintaining the space at the back of the mouth with an 'inside smile'.

5. Using the following word list create a gentle onset by bringing the vocal folds together very gently so as not to damage them. Linger momentarily on the /h/ at the start of the following words and then drop the /h/ and say the word:

h~able	*able*	*h~over*	*over*
h~increase	*increase*	*h~ill*	*ill*
h~india	*india*	*h~older*	*older*
h~open	*open*	*h~eat*	*eat*
h~up	*up*	*h~until*	*until*
h~even	*even*	*h~enjoy*	*enjoy*
h~attitude	*attitude*	*h~andy*	*Andy*
h~ideal	*ideal*	*h~accident*	*accident*
h~instant	*instant*	*h~environment*	*environment*

6. Use the following sentences to practice the onset of vowels. Begin with /h/ in the first instance if necessary.

Ian is ever the enthusiast.
Oliver always overestimates other individuals' interest in igloos.
Angela always answers eventually.
Ivan investigates important issues and is an advocate for education.
Important enemy information infiltrated the infantry.
Ultimately the umbrellas were assigned to the athletes.
Unable to alter the opulent orange eider overcoat, Amy offered to ex-
*   change it.*

7. Speak the following with a raised volume, applying the /h/ initially:

Anthony, ask Olivia for the art assignment please.
Everybody, I am asking for your attention.
Ethan and Amanda, over here immediately please.
All athletes attending acrobatic appraisals please gather in the arena.
At the end of the exercise everyone should help to gather the equipment.

Muscularity and articulation

When working on your own muscularity and when addressing muscularity issues in the classroom remember that work on muscles is most effective:

- when relaxation and breathing exercises precede muscularity exercises;
- when due attention is paid to the articulators, with a sense of awareness of the intrinsic movement of each;
- when exercises are undertaken at an easy pace initially – the pace can be increased as dexterity and muscularity improves;
- when negative patterns are changed and replaced with more effective patterns;
- with increased mobility of the articulators;
- with visual and kinesthetic feedback – this can be achieved by the use of a mirror, cell/mobile phone camera;
- when minimal effort is used to produce easy flowing co-ordination in the articulators – speech should look comfortable and easy;
- if emotional tension held in the jaw and the root of the tongue can be recognized and monitored;
- if there is understanding and awareness of the role played by the breath in the articulation of consonants;
- when exercising with rhythm and range – avoid getting stuck in a monotonous and mechanical pattern of delivery;
- when words are connected to meaning at all times;
- when an uninhibited desire to communicate is present so that easy, energized flexible speech is more easily achieved;
- if exercise is regular and routines are established and continued;
- if undertaken in an accurate and specific manner; and
- if practice material is carefully selected and is age-appropriate.

When working on your own muscularity and when addressing muscularity issues in the classroom remember that work on muscles is of limited effectiveness:

- if excessive or undue tension is present in the articulators;
- if allied head and shoulder tension is present;
- if habitual postural tension gives rise to the tongue being carried high in the mouth;
- if minimal jaw opening produces subsequent tension in the oropharynx and tongue root;
- if breath is held while exercising;
- if undertaken too quickly in the first instance;
- if muscles are forced or over-stretched;
- if exercise is only sporadic and regular routines are not established;
- if undertaken in a generalized and non-specific manner; or
- if exercises are undertaken by rote and without a connection between words, thought and meaning.

Before embarking on exercises for muscularity it is important to release tension and stress. Yawning and stretching is a beneficial form of exercise to precede work on muscularity.

Yawning and stretching

- Yawning and stretching releases tension and stimulates energy, and should be utilized at points throughout a session.
- The yawn opens up the oral space, stretches the facial muscles, lifts the soft palate, releases the jaw.
- It is an excellent way in which to release tension in the oropharynx.
- It also provides extra oxygen and is energizing.
- The yawn should be enjoyed, not stifled or suppressed.

Exercises for the jaw

The mouth is the only truly moveable resonator and it is important for it to be relaxed and flexible in order for voice and speech to be resonant and free. Any release exercises should be done from the 'hinge' of the jaw and not from the front of the mouth.

1. Yawning is an excellent way to release tension in the jaw and pharynx, and the release of tension increases muscularity. Do not stifle yawns; enjoy them.

2. Imagine that you are chewing a piece of toffee. Use the whole mouth space and jaw. To avoid this becoming a way of inadvertently increasing tension in the jaw, work with a relaxed, almost slow motion energy that aims to stretch the strap muscles of the jaw.

3. Imagine that you have small springs between your molars, which do not allow your teeth to touch, so that the result of attempting to bring the teeth together would be that they spring away from each other. This springing movement also increases the length of the jaw muscles.

4. Place your hands on either side of the face and gently stroke the jaw downwards. Allow the mouth to open as the hands move down the face. Keep the jaw loose, free, and mobile.

5. Holding on to the chin with the thumb and fingers of one hand, tip the head backwards, as if you were able to lift the upper jaw. Create space in the mouth and between the teeth. Keep the tongue relaxed.

Exercises for the lips

1. Lips need to be exercised in order to keep the muscles capable of making firm explosive sounds flexibly and without creating neck and jaw tension. First, purse the lips forward and then spread them suddenly into a broad smile. It is important to be aware of the muscles used in the two activities.

2. Curl the upper lip up towards the nose. Curl the lower lip down towards the chin. Purse the lips and then open and close the pursed lips in an action that resembles the mouth of a goldfish.

3. Try balancing a pencil on the upper lip.

4. Blow up the cheeks and then, using your fingers, 'pop' the cheeks, producing a sound as the air explodes through the lips.

5. Produce an exploding /b/ sound using the lips. Increase this to three /b/s followed by a vowel, e.g., /b/b/bah/. Do the same with /p/. Follow this with vowels that end on a /b/, e.g./oob/ and /ohb/, and with /p/, e.g., /oop/ and /ohp/.

6. Working on the sound /w/ exercises the lips:

   Whether the weather be fine
   or whether the weather be not.
   Whether the weather be cold
   or whether the weather be hot.
   We'll weather the weather
   whether we like it or not.

7. Speak these sentences accentuating the movement of the lips:

   Patricia and Pamela are particular about their potted plants.
   Can you remember when we two were wed?
   Whistle for William when he is out on the moors with Monty.
   Barney blotted his copybook when he bungled the booking for Peter.
   Many mischievous monkeys perpetually munch bananas and peanuts.
   Brilliant Beatrice beat the boys at backgammon.

Exercises for the tongue

1. Extend the tongue out of the mouth. The tongue tip should make a thin, pointed shape. Follow this by spreading the sides of the tongue so that it becomes wider and flatter. Keep alternating these positions. If necessary, place two fingers either side of the tongue as a 'guide' to encourage a sideways spread of the tongue.

2. Tuck the tongue tip behind the lower front teeth and flatten the blade of the tongue in the mouth. Alter the mass of the tongue by bunching it forward and out of the mouth while maintaining contact with the lower front teeth with the tongue tip.

3. The following exercise aims to stretch the middle of the tongue. Place the tip behind the lower front teeth and then bunch the mid-

dle of the tongue forward and out of the mouth. Hold the stretched position for a few seconds and then release.

4. Extend the tongue out of the mouth, starting with a large circular movement and decreasing until the circle is very small. Reverse this by starting with a small circle and increasing until a large circle is achieved.

5. Stick the tongue out of the mouth with the sides folded upward so that the tongue forms a funnel shape. Next flatten the sides so that the tongue is wide and flat. Repeat this exercise, alternately funneling and flattening the tongue.

6. Extending the tongue with tongue tip pointed, use it like a pen to 'draw' a picture of a house, a seascape, a boat, or to 'write' the title of a book, a film, or a TV programme.

7. Move the tongue rapidly in and out of the mouth, rather as a cat does when it laps milk.

8. Roll the tip and body of the tongue backward into the mouth towards the soft palate and then quickly flick it out again, rather like a lizard or chameleon when catching a fly.

9. Extend the tongue and try to touch your nose with the tip of your tongue.

10. Place a straw in the funnel in the middle of the tongue and blow down the straw. Once this is established remove the straw. Continue to blow (breathe out) down the funnel.

11. Using the straw placed in the middle of the tongue, blow bubbles into a glass one-third filled with water.

12. The tongue needs to be exercised so that it is capable of flexible movement without tension. To start, simply stretch the tongue as far out of the mouth as you can and then allow it to relax back into the mouth, leaving the tip touching the lower front teeth.

13. Lift the tongue to the ridge behind the upper teeth and explode the consonant sequence /d/d/d/d/ and /t/t/t/t/. Lift the tongue and form an /l/, then precede the /l/ by a series of vowels, e.g., /eel/ /ool/

/ahl/ /ohl/ /awl/. Use a series of words containing /l/ to exercise the tongue; these can be done with children, asking them to supply the words, e.g., *lorry, land, light, cool, feel, hold, golden, lazy, languid.*

14. Repeat the above exercise using an /r/ in place of the /l/. Continue on to words such as *run, rowing, rugged, ripple, rusty* and phrases such as *red roses, running riot, real rabbits, rabid rodents, road runner, rusty railings,* and *rhubarb rhubarb.*

15. Work on the medial /r/ with words such as *lorry, Larry, tomorrow, carry, sorrow, merry, worry, terrible,* and *terrific.* The medial /r/ can also be exercised by singing the traditional rhyme

> *Row, row, row your boat,*
> *Gently down the stream.*
> *Merrily, merrily, merrily, merrily*

The blended /r/ can be exercised by these words and phrases: *train, trap, brain, broad, drain, drape, pray, prime, crime, create, great, grotesque, street, straight,* and *Craig crushes grown gremlins, Trevor dreams of dreadful dragons, Brian breaks trains and tractors.*

Exercises for the soft palate

1. In order to identify the soft palate, sound a sharp /k/ and /g/ several times, then add a vowel to the consonant producing /kah/, /koh/, /kaw/ and /gah/, /goh/, /gaw/.

2. Speak these words, sustaining the /ng/ sound at the end: *ring, thing, sing, rang, bang, pang, king.* Then repeat the /ng/ sound and open sharply into a vowel /ng-ah/, /ng-oh/, /ng-aw/.

3. Create the sound of a siren, using the sounds /ng-ah/ng-oh/ changing pitch as you do so. Repeat several times.

4. Repeat the consonants /k/ and /g/ several times in isolation, and then repeat /k/ and open to the vowels /ah/, /aw/, /oh/, /oo/, /ay/,/ ee/ and /ow/. Repeat the exercise with /g/ followed by each of these vowels: /ah/, /aw/, /oh/, /oo/, /ay/,/ee/ and /ow/.

5.   Speak these sentences:

A king carried crates of cabbages across a crooked court.

A skunk sat on a stump. The skunk thunk the stump stunk and the stump
    thunk the skunk stunk.

Carly cannot carry Luca to the car.

Can you catch a kookaburra Kevin?

Garron gives gifts to Krystal.

Cameron carries grapes in a crate to Margaret.

Christopher, can you recount the capitals of countries such as Canada,
    Kuwait, Croatia, and Cuba?

Kingfishers catch colourful creatures.

Final consonants

The following text is useful to increase attention to these:

As I was going to St Ives,
I met a man with seven wives.
Each wife had seven sacks,
Each sack had seven cats,
Each cat had seven kits:
Kits, cats, sacks, and wives,
How many were there going to St Ives?

Complex consonant clusters

These sounds are important for professional voice users who need dexterity and precision for clarity. Actors need to be able to produce the full spectrum of sounds depending on what is required for a specific role. They therefore need to be flexible and capable of executing any articulatory demands. A tendency in contemporary speech is to allow the /s/ to become a /sh/ resulting in *shtreet, shtride* etc. This should be avoided.

1.   Words beginning with /str/:

straddle   *strain*   *straggle*

straight	*stray*	*strata*
stride	*stroke*	*strong*
strict	*strut*	*stripe*
struck	*strudel*	*strictly*
strongly	*strip*	*streamer*

2. Words with /st/ at the end:

thirst	*ghost*	*worst*
first	*just*	*wrist*
post	*bust*	*pest*
rest	*must*	*hoist*

3. Words with /sts/ at the end:

pests	*posts*	*roasts*
hosts	*masts*	*priests*
firsts	*chests*	*lists*
thrusts	*boasts*	*toasts*

Muscularity in text

Additional muscularity not only increases clarity and volume but also connects words with their inherent meaning and power. An excellent and enriching way of exercising the muscles of speech is to work on extant material. Tongue twisters are useful and can be fun, but they can be ill-advised if they are articulated with tension or merely 'rattled off' without being related to meaning. There is much wonderfully structured and well honed verse available, offering not just a muscular exercise, but stimulation of the imagination and in addition, demanding commitment to rhythm and phrasing. The benefits of using verse are numerous because these passages increase vocabulary, stimulate ideas and discussion, and offer the experience of speaking out loud and exploring the power of language. Verse also has marked rhythm, which connects the speaker with the syllabic energy of language and the ways in which this energy and the heightened language affect the speaker and the audience. As well as verse it is useful to work on well structured prose and political speeches. These exercise the speaker's ability to share stories and, in the case of political speeches, to persuade and explore the power of words. They are also a useful aid in history classes.

1.   Speak the following text exploring the dynamic of the language.

> *You lie, in faith, for you are call'd plain Kate,*
> *And bonny Kate, and sometimes Kate the curst:*
> *But, Kate, the prettiest Kate in Christendom,*
> *Kate of Kate Hall, my super-dainty Kate,*
> *Take this of me, Kate of my consolation.*
>
> William Shakespeare, *The Taming of the Shrew* (Act II, scene I)

2.   When speaking this poem, articulate precisely, dexterously and quietly while keeping the rhythm. Avoid forcing the energy or raising the volume.

> *Stone walls do not a prison make,*
> *Nor iron bars a cage;*
> *Minds innocent and quiet take*
> *That for an hermitage;*
> *If I have freedom in my love*
> *And in my soul am free,*
> *Angels alone, that soar above,*
> *Enjoy such liberty.*
>
> Richard Lovelace, *To Althea from Prison* (1642).

3.   In the following text feel the contact between the lips in words such as bleeding, piece, butchers etc., the contact between the back of the tongue and soft palate in curse, costly and groaning etc., and the flexibility of the tongue in tide, times and revenge, etc. Explore the connection between the sounds and the content and emotion of the passage.

O, pardon me, thou bleeding piece of earth,

That I am meek and gentle with these butchers!

Thou art the ruins of the noblest man

That ever lived in the tide of times.

Woe to the hand that shed this costly blood!

Over thy wounds now do I prophesy,—

Which, like dumb mouths, do ope their ruby lips,

To beg the voice and utterance of my tongue—

A curse shall light upon the limbs of men;

Domestic fury and fierce civil strife

Shall cumber all the parts of Italy;

Blood and destruction shall be so in use

And dreadful objects so familiar

That mothers shall but smile when they behold

Their infants quarter'd with the hands of war;

All pity choked with custom of fell deeds:

And Caesar's spirit, ranging for revenge,

With Ate by his side come hot from hell,

Shall in these confines with a monarch's voice

Cry 'Havoc,' and let slip the dogs of war;

That this foul deed shall smell above the earth

With carrion men, groaning for burial.

William Shakespeare, *Julius Caesar* by (Act III, scene I)

Syllables and stress patterns and their role in clarity

Many contemporary speakers pay little attention to the value of syllables in speech. Modern speech is often elided or contracted in an effort to make it sound friendly or relaxed. Equally, haste can be the cause of not giving syllables their appropriate value. Many people feel, often correctly, that they are being over-aggressive or pedantic if they give full value to syllables. This problem is avoided by not over-stressing and using both the stressed and the unstressed syllables in words.

Over-stressing means stressing every word or every syllable in a word and not observing the unstressed syllable, and it is this that sounds pedantic and monotonous because it removes the music from the language. It is natural for native English speakers to observe the unstressed sound in, for example, the phrase 'a man and a woman' rather than the stressed '*a* man and *a* woman'. Equally the spelled 'a' in the word 'woman' is not given full stress. We don't say wo-***man***.

Enjoyment of the musicality of words gives them clarity and muscular energy, which is bound up with defining the syllables and committing to the consonants. As well as defining the syllable, it is important to release the rhythm by stressing the appropriate syllable.

First language speakers assimilate the correct stress pattern in words in their native tongue, but speakers of English as a second language often find this aspect of the language difficult and frustrating because there are no concrete rules. One of the most frequent problems in audibility for second language English speakers is incorrect syllabic stress. Notice how changing the stress in the words 'allow' and 'control' (from unstress/stress to stress/unstress) makes the word difficult to recognize.

An appreciation of syllables is particularly important in teaching because it is in the classroom that students are often introduced to a word for the first time. Clearly enunciating syllables assists audibility. Second language speakers should ask colleagues for help with identifying the stress in unfamiliar words.

As well as knowing where the stress falls, it is important to enjoy the contact with the consonants rather than to smooth over and minimize them. Consider the number of syllables in these words:

> *library*
> *escalation*
> *discombobulate*
> *January*

February

articulate

procrastination

vulnerable

multiplication

eradicate

escalator

explanatory.

Giving value to the syllables is a simple and effective way of increasing audibility. Although elision or contraction is usually acceptable in conversational speech, once there is distance to cover and information to exchange, success is more likely if the syllables are given their natural weight.

The muscular engagement required enhances the articulation of the word as well as releasing the rhythm and impetus. This avoids monotony that often results from a lack of syllabic energy, and monotonous speech can be difficult to understand.

Speakers who are rushing will invariably compromise the syllabic value of words as will those who 'shy away' from the physical and mental commitment to the word. This may be because they do not wish to appear forceful or encroach on the personal space of the listener, or because they are over-familiar with the material. Easy confident muscular engagement with syllables gives the audience a sense that the speaker 'owns' the space as well as the subject matter.

A word of caution

Avoid stressing the 'weak' or unstressed syllables because this will result in a staccato sound that is as monotonous as not articulating or stressing the appropriate syllables. It may also be perceived as being over-bearing and pedantic. It is important to balance syllabic value with the music and rhythm of the language.

Exercises for identifying stressed and unstressed syllables

Speak the words below and stress only those syllables that require it. Notice the rhythm that results. Try giving all the syllables equal value; in this way you will hear how very robotic you sound. If English is your second language these words might be difficult so ask a colleague for help with which syllables to stress.

to-day	*es-ca-la-tor*	*imm-i-gra-tion*
Fa-cul-ty	*hos-pit-al*	*com-pu-ter*
ag-i-tate	*Dim-i-tri*	*Shos-ta-kov-ich*
claus-tro-pho-bic	*ec-cen-tri-ci-ty*	*ac-cel-er-ate*
per-pen-dic-u-lar	*mus-cu-lar-i-ty*	*Rim-sky-Kor-sa-kov*
in-teg-ri-ty	*in-ter-pre-tive*	*his-tri-on-ics*
the-a-tri-cal	*al-pha-bet-i-cal*	*his-tor-i-cal*

The British Council has a *Teaching English* website that may be of interest, especially to speakers of English as a second language. Details can be found at the end of the chapter.

The unstressed neutral vowel

Naturally rhythmical speakers instinctively know when not to stress a syllable. Once again, second language speakers may find themselves encountering difficulties and tending to stress too many. The English language is one of both 'stress and unstress' and the neutral vowel is a great aid to easy rhythm. The sound (not the spelling) of the neutral is 'a' (as in above) and may be found in words such as *father, mother, sister, brother, anger, folder* etc., and at the beginning of the following words: *abundant, ago*. The sound can be spelt in many ways, such as 'er' in mother, 'a' in allow. It is also found in the middle of words such as *corporation* and *coronation* – spelt with 'o'.

The same applies to the definite article /the/. 'The' only becomes /thee/ when it precedes a vowel as in the following examples, /thee egg/, /thee ostrich/, /thee inkpot/. Both first and second language speakers will often 'over-correct' this sound and over-stress in an attempt to sound clear and well spoken. Natural sounding speech with flow and rhythm should always be the goal. Second language speakers often find English confusing because it has only five written vowels, but these have many sounds, approximately 24 in all, depending on accent and dialect.

Chapter outline

- Posture and posture exercises
- Shoulders and shoulder exercises
- Neck and neck exercises
- Relaxation and relaxation exercises
- Breathing
- Are you a breath-holder?
- Exercises for releasing held breath
- Resonance and resonance exercises
- Forward placement and exercises for forward placement
- De-constriction and onset of the note
- Muscularity and articulation
- Muscularity and articulation exercises
- Muscularity in text exercises
- Syllables and stress patterns and their role in clarity
- The unstressed neutral vowel

References and further reading

British Council. *Teaching English*. Available at: <http://www.teachingenglish.org.uk/> [Accessed August 2017].

12

Further exercises for pitch range, vocal variety, and speech making

As well as offering exercises for development of pitch range and vocal variety, this chapter also offers strategies for speech making and provides several exercise and warm-up routines.

For educators, a varied pitch range and vocal variety adds expressivity and is an asset that allows classes or audiences to better engage with, and remember, what is being said.

When talking about pitch, what is actually being described in very simple terms is how high or how low the note is when produced by the vocal folds. Pitch changes occur naturally throughout life from childhood to adulthood to old age. In general, men's voices are lower in pitch than women's but in some instances, expected pitch changes do not occur and individuals do not have access to a pitch range that is appropriate to their age and gender. Pitch range refers to the variety of pitch which is within the vocal repertoire of an individual. Pitch movement, when it occurs within a word, is known as inflection while pitch movement over a series of phrases or sentences is known as intonation.

Someone who speaks in a monotone would be considered to have a narrow range whereas someone who modulates the voice and encompasses a variety of pitches, both high and low, is deemed to have a wide range.

When working on your own pitch range and when addressing pitch-related issues in the classroom, remember that work on pitch is most effective:

- when preliminary work is undertaken on range;
- when there has been an assessment of vocal range both sung and spoken;
- if carryover from exercises into conversational use is the goal;
- if range and flexibility within and around the pitch is explored;
- if self-monitoring and auditory awareness of the new pitch is achieved;
- if family, friends, and colleagues can be persuaded to 'accept' the new pitch;
- if the individual works towards achieving a pitch range which is perceived as appropriate to age and gender;
- if exercises are undertaken in a playful manner – all drama exercises should support this work; and
- if the vocal pitch responds naturally to changes in thought and emotion.

This final point can be practiced by reading poetry or reading to an audience (storytelling), or by role-playing a news reader or reporter.

When working on your own pitch and when addressing pitch-related issues in the classroom remember that work on pitch is of limited effectiveness:

- if there is tension present in the muscles which will limit the range and flexibility of the vocal folds and compromise the pitch;
- if too little time is spent on identifying the habitual pitch range;
- if too little time is spent on exploring the full and natural vocal range;
- if inhibition or habit leads to monotonous delivery in everyday conversation;
- if the voice is forced into an artificially high or low pitch; or
- if the voice regularly repeats a specific pitch pattern.

Preliminary exercises for range

Exercises for range will have appeared in other chapters as part of developing volume and resonance. Range is more evident in relaxed voices so endeavour to have fun with these exercises which for some may be daunting or exposing.

Sliding and gliding

Use the whole body and move whenever possible during these exercises.

1. Sirening: using the sound /n/ (and imitating the noise of a police siren) describe a vocal circle that begins between the shoulder blades and 'slide' the sound over the top of the head and face. Keeping the sound moving, return to the starting point along an imaginary circular trajectory. This should be easy as long as you keep it playful and do not try to push. You will not hurt the voice in this way. The same can be done with the /ng/ sound (in *song*) and the /m/ /v/ and /z/.

2. Sliding: stretching up with hands in the air, allow the spine to bend over, one vertebra at a time, until you are bent over at the waist. As you do so make the sound of a vowel, such as /oo/ /ay/ /aw/ or /ah/. Make the vowel last as long as the journey from the extended stretch to the bent spine. This exercise can be done in reverse, starting the sound on the floor and sliding it upwards. Some people find this direction easier; others find it more difficult. Eventually both will be possible. If you find the onset of the vowel difficult precede it with an /m/.

3. Bowling: using the arm to bowl, imagine the ball is the sound /m/ and as it leaves your hand lift the sound up and over the space almost in an arc. Open to the vowel /ah/ halfway through the arc and sustain the sound until it 'lands' on the ground. Do this in slow motion so that it blends from the /m/ into the /ah/ smoothly as it arcs through the air.

4. (a) Glide from chest to mouth: make /ah/, producing chest resonance. Feel the vibration by placing your hand on your chest. Make

an /aw/, being aware of the resonance in the mouth. Notice how the lips form a megaphone shape.

(b)   Begin by patting the chest while sounding /mah/ and feel the vibrations. Glide the /ah/ vowel into an /aw/ in the mouth, slurring from one sound to another, e.g., /mah ... aw/

(c)   Repeat the exercise beginning with the /aw/ resonating in the mouth and then glide this sound upwards into an /ee/. The glide from the /aw/ to the /ee/ should be relaxed and effortless, and the overall balance of one sound moving from one space to another should be maintained. In all these exercises the smooth continuum of sound is worked for, and any feeling of pushed or strangulated sounds should be avoided. If a 'crack' in the flow of sound develops, just go slowly back over that area in the range. Using the hand or arm to describe the movement is often an effective aid to developing flexibility of the voice.

5.   Fire engine/ambulance siren: using /ng ... ah//ng ... ah//ng ... ah/, create movement between head and chest resonance. This exercise explores the vocal range and extends the extremes of pitch and resonance. The dual-pitch siren is used for different vehicles in different cities, so the title of this exercise may not be correct for everyone, but can be adapted.

6.   Slurring and singing: using a piece of text or the lyrics of a song (just a few lines), slur the voice drunkenly and smoothly through the whole range. Try a line sung to a made-up tune. Speak it to that tune. Omit the tune but keep the movement in the voice.

Playful range exercises

It is important to 'play' and not to strive for perfection because this usually results in creating tension rather than releasing it.

1.   Draw a wavy line and trace this pattern with your finger as you sound /oo/ moving up and down your range.

2.   If you or someone else can play the piano, sing scales, exploring your range on different vowels.

3.   'Sing' phrases or sentences in an 'operatic' voice. The verse in the following exercise can be used for this. Keep the exercise playful.

4.   Using these words deliberately move (or preferably slur) the voice from your lowest notes to your highest:

Since there's no help, come let us kiss and part,—
Nay I have done, you get no more of me;
And I am glad, yea, glad with all my heart,
That thus so cleanly I myself can free.

From: Michael Drayton, Loves Farewell (circa 1619)

5.   Using the word *bubble*, begin with a low pitched, large 'gloopy' bubble and raise the pitch as bubbles get smaller and lighter. Use the body to help create the image.

6.   In pairs, imagine you are out of doors on a mountain, on a beach, or in a field, then call to a friend to 'Come this way' gesturing with your hand as you call. The friend should reply 'Are you sure, I thought it was that way'. Keep moving a few steps further apart after every exchange. Notice how the voice needs more breath support and range as the distance between the pair widens.

Exercises for establishing pitch range

1.   Sing, chant, or hum on /ah/ up and down a scale – keep it playful. Note the top and bottom pitch. If this proves too difficult start 'as low as possible' and go up 'as high as possible'. If this is still difficult for those with a very restricted range, start on a note that is comfortable, again singing, chanting or humming on /ah/, and see how much 'movement' there is around the note (this entails singing, chanting, or humming a note slightly above or below).

If 'movement' is very limited initially, work on the exercises gently but regularly, extending pitch range little by little.

2. Many words encourage the use of a high or low pitch because of their meaning and associated sound. The following word lists are useful to encourage pitch change. Although this exercise may seem rather unnatural, using contrastive pairs of words is an excellent way in which to encourage variety of pitch. It should be approached in a playful manner:

High pitch	Low pitch
ding	dong
crash	tinkle
clash	zing
growl	hiss
bellow	shriek
guffaw	giggle
cough	sneeze
groan	exclaim
rough	smooth
light	dark
giggle	sigh
high	low
playful	serious
mountains	plains
smile	frown
hissed	droned
jump	dive
up	down
jovial	grumpy
lithe	sluggish
ceiling	floor
treble	bass
bubble	swirl
soft	hard

hopeful	*disappointed*
air	*earth*
comedy	*tragedy*
play	*work*
holiday	*school*
delight	*dismay*
tip	*base*
tinkled	*crashed*
excited	*bored*

3. Once effective use of high and low pitch has been established in sin-
    gle words, move on to using them in sentences. Changes in tone will
    also be noted, particularly if the approach is playful and uninhibited.
    Explore higher pitch using these sentences:

The sky was shining with millions of twinkling stars.
The sun danced and sparkled on the water.
The balloon floated up into the clear, blue sky.
The tiny kitten climbed to the very top of the tree.
The wind took the kite soaring high up into the sky.
The wind blew the hat into the air.
The birds cheeped and fluttered in the trees.
The ball bounced higher and higher and into the net.
The girl had never felt so happy and excited.
She laughed and laughed with happiness.
The baby chuckled and gurgled with delight.
The teenagers shrieked with joy as they ran out of school.
The cork popped and flew up out of the champagne bottle.
The sound of the choristers could be heard resounding in the church.
The church bells pealed out a joyful sound.
The girls giggled and tried to suppress their mirth.

4.   Sentences for exploring low pitch:

The news was full of gloom.
Slowly and quietly the burglar crept around the building in the moonlight.
The man was a prisoner in the dark, dreary dungeon.
Threw the prisoner into the cell.
Deep in the dark forest the girl was lost.
There was no way out of the tunnel.
The pilot parachuted slowly to earth as his plane crashed.
The basking shark swam around in the murky waters.
The miner went down the lift shaft into the depths of the earth.
The boy trudged slowly home in the dark.
The man was slumped at the side of the road, exhausted.
The sun sank slowly in the west and there was darkness.
The woman was taken into hospital ill and dying.
The man had a gruff and angry voice.

5.   Using sentences which are questions is a good way of raising pitch. It is important to ask the question from the start of the sentence not just on the final word:

How did you do that?
Where is the bottle of pills?
Is it true there was a storm last night?
Can you help me, please?
What is your opinion of this?
Which road should we take?
Has the last train gone?
Is that your sister over there?
Who is going to open this gate?
What time does this shop open?
Have you any idea what time it is?
Did you hear about the accident?

Was this starting at eight or nine o'clock?
Does it matter which way up this goes?
Who did you say was in this play?
Is your brother that man with the grey hair?

6.   Using the months of the year, alternate high and low pitches: *January* will be said with a high pitch, *February* with a low pitch, *March* with a high pitch, and so on. Repeat the exercise, starting with *January* on a low pitch.

7.   An alternative exercise is to use a sequence of numbers (begin at one), gradually rising in pitch with each one. This exercise may be practiced in reverse, so that the first number is on a high pitch and each successive number gets lower. The exercise above may then be developed so that short sentences are used, again with each successive word becoming higher and higher or lower and lower in pitch, as appropriate. The following sentences can be used:

I can climb higher and higher.
I got more and more excited as the orchestra started to play.
I became more and more depressed as the story went on.
Alice fell, down, down, down into the rabbit hole.
I can jump higher and higher and higher on the trampoline.
I slipped and the ball dropped.
Jack and Jill went up the hill, right to the very top.
The kite climbed higher and higher into the sky, swooped, dived, and
    floated slowly down to earth.

8.   Use higher and lower pitches appropriately in the following sentences. Explore the drama and do not be concerned if you sound unnatural at this point:

The news was full of gloom as rumours of war began to spread, but it
    was a bright spring morning and the church bells pealed out a joyful
    sound.

While the wind howled in the trees and the snow began to fall, in the
cottage, by the fireside, the baby chuckled and gurgled with delight.
The dank cave was cold and gloomy, and we had become very despondent
when someone suddenly shouted, 'I can see a glimmer of daylight, run
quickly everyone, this way!'

9. For movement up and down the scale try the following exercise.
    Use the hand to manipulate an imaginary yo-yo. Using the sound
    /oo/ move the pitch up and down the scale following the movement
    of the yo-yo. When the yo-yo is high the pitch is high when the
    yo-yo is low the pitch is low. Allow the voice to glide effortlessly
    between the notes. Then take the yo-yo to greater extremes of height
    and depths, letting the voice follow. Never push the sound; keep it
    relaxed and flowing. This may be tried with other vowel sounds: /ay/,
    /ee/ and /ai/.

10. Speak these sentences using as much innuendo or sarcasm as you
    can:

    Hello where have you been?
    Of course I believe you, who wouldn't.
    Really, how amazing.
    Facts? Who needs facts!
    Late? No, you are never late!
    Well, what do you expect?
    Surprise, surprise.

11. Now apply the yo-yo exercise to this line of prose:

    Why are you walking when the weather's wild?

    Do not play 'safe'; allow the voice to sound uncontrolled and pos-
    sibly silly. Variety and movement in the pitch range should occur in
    individual words as well as in the sentence. Other lines to use are:

Silly Susan sleeps in solitary silence.

Have you seen my sister Jean?

You and I are really running round and round in circles.

When the east wind howls and the waves are wild you ought to hide inside.

Vocal variety

When working on your own vocal variety and when addressing monotony-related issues in the classroom, remember that work on variety is most effective:

- when a link is developed between the mind, emotion, and language;
- when appropriate material is used to gently encourage and extend vocal variety; for example, poetry, descriptive and humorous prose, exciting narrative, and dramatic excerpts;
- when awareness of the dynamics of words is encouraged so that language becomes alive rather than simply printed symbols of communication;
- when using verse and well honed literature which helps to develop an awareness of the rhythm of words and which in turn may be assimilated into spontaneous usage in conversational speech;
- if an appreciation of the use of image in language has been developed, as this aids the development of vibrant thought-related speech;
- if imagination/visualization of language is exercised so that the dynamic of the spoken word matches the emotional content of the language;
- when stamping, clapping, dancing, and moving while speaking is used to release rhythm and dynamics in language; and
- when role play is explored in order to move away from predictable or habitual vocal patterns – assuming a character can be most valuable in voice work as it gives freedom to explore alternative usage of voice.

When working on your own vocal variety and when addressing monotony-related issues in the classroom, remember that work on variety is of limited effectiveness:

- if tension restricts and suppresses the pitch range;
- if speech patterns are imposed or imitated;
- if uninteresting, banal 'chew rag' material is used, as it will reduce interest and commitment by the speaker; or
- if emotionally charged material is used without proper consideration of mood and emotional status.

Exercises for varying intonation and inflection

1. Using only *yes* and *no*, try to convey enthusiasm, boredom, certainty, and doubt when answering the following questions:

   Is your favourite composer Mozart?
   Have you done your homework?
   Is your favourite food scrambled egg?
   Are you going to Los Angeles?
   Did you see Dan take the bike?
   Would you like some cake?
   Can I ask you a delicate question?
   Will you be home by ten?

2. Using intonation to express the meaning in brackets, answer the question: *Do you like this wallpaper?* with the following sentences:

   I'm not sure (doubt)
   Certainly not (certainty)
   I can't take this question seriously (amusement)
   What does it matter what I think (boredom)
   Why are you asking? (irritation)
   I can't stand that colour (disgust)
   Why ask my opinion? (questioning)

Monitor the way in which the voice changes in pitch, inflects and alters in pace in these differing responses.

3. Answer the question *Are you sure you know what to do?* Respond with a *yes* to convey:

Of course I do (disdain)
No, not really (uncertainty)
I'll go crazy if I'm asked again (long-suffering)
Yes, and now I must go (definite)
Are you suggesting I don't (annoyance)?
Why, don't you? (sarcasm)

4. See how many different ways the following words can be said and notice the movement of the voice as it inflects in order to convey meaning: *oh, hello, never, eventually, sorry, thank you, when?, really, why?, honestly.*

5. Use the days of the week, the months of the year, and so on to convey meaning, for example:

- Explain how to bake a cake using only the days of the week as words.
- Teach a geography lesson using *January, February, March,* and so on.
- Sell fruit on a market stall using *A, B, C,* and so on.
- Preach a sermon using the numbers one to five.
- Describe an emergency using the surnames Smith, Jones, and White.
- Give directions from the town centre to the railway station using only vowels.
- Give directions from the town centre to the railway station using only consonants.

NB: It is very important with all these exercises to have a clear intention of what is to be said before starting.

337

6. In these sentences, place the subordinate clause on a higher or lower pitch so that both parts of the main (or principal clause) are connected:

   John, my elder brother, is a fireman.
   The flowers, the daisies not the roses, are from my garden.
   Yesterday, which was really hot, we took the children swimming.
   My mother, in her youth, travelled extensively.
   Joe and Stephen, Joe is a doctor, both play tennis.
   The central station, there are two in the town, is on Main Street.
   Mrs Ryan, who runs the corner shop, is originally from Australia.

7. Try to find a physical action/gesture to express the dynamics of words such as: *thump, thrust, rumble, quake, pull, push, press, cuddle, clutch, grab, climb, shake, dash, dig, wobble, churn, flick, grapple.*

   Make gestures larger than life and do not try to be too literal. Mime along with the words, fitting gesture to word wherever possible.

8. Using only nonsense words create the following scenarios:

   - Two long-standing friends meet after some time apart and exchange news.
   - Bringing an injured animal to the vet.
   - Two political rivals argue over the establishment of a new highway.
   - Discussion about a television 'soap'.
   - Returning a faulty item to a shop and complaining to the manager.

9. Working with melodramatic scenarios is a very effective way of developing and extending range, intonation, pause and pace. Work on melodrama should be approached with a playful attitude. It is equally important that the environment created is a positive one that promotes the freedom to experiment and risk.

A melodramatic scenario will allow the freedom to play and to go 'over the top' vocally, experiencing variety of range and volume. Gradually the exaggerated vocal range can be toned down and a more natural quality achieved, but the experience of variety is retained.

This short duologue can be used to develop a melodramatic scene, or can just be explored to extend vocal delivery:

A: *Where has he gone?*

B: *Who?*

A: *Joseph.*

B: *That way, I think.*

A: *Do you know why?*

B: *He refused to say.*

A: *Oh, this is terrible!*

B: *Why?*

A: *I think he is vile.*

B: *I rather like him.*

A: *I am sorry to say it but the man's a rogue!*

B: *Oh, please don't say that, I lent him some money!*

10. Using this extract from Charles Dickens's *A Christmas Carol*, use changes in pitch to convey the characters of Scrooge, the boy, and the narrator. (NB: 'Walk-er' is an exclamation of disbelief.)

"Hallo, my fine fellow!"

"Hallo!" returned the boy.

"Do you know the Poulterer's, in the next street but one, at the corner?" Scrooge inquired.

"I should hope I did," replied the lad.

"An intelligent boy!" said Scrooge. "A remarkable boy! Do you know whether they've sold the prize Turkey that was hanging up there?
— Not the little prize Turkey: the big one?"

"What, the one as big as me?" returned the boy.

"What a delightful boy!" said Scrooge. "It's a pleasure to talk to him.
Yes, my buck!"
"It's hanging there now," replied the boy.
"Is it?" said Scrooge. "Go and buy it."
"Walk-er!" exclaimed the boy.
"No, no," said Scrooge, "I am in earnest. Go and buy it, and tell 'em
to bring it here, that I may give them the direction where to take it.
Come back with the man, and I'll give you a shilling. Come back
with him in less than five minutes and I'll give you half-a-crown!"

A note on pause and pace

Two non-vocal elements that add variety to speech are pause and pace. They create a sense of anticipation and movement to communication.

Pauses are valuable in creating anticipation and atmosphere, and when wishing to emphasize important facts and phrases. Pauses in the wrong place can break the sense of a phrase and confuse the listener.

A change to a faster pace in an exciting passage will add to the experience of the listener; slowing down the pace can suggest a conclusion, while a pace that is too regular becomes monotonous and can cause the listener to disengage or lose interest. As always, the advice is to be guided by the meaning. The more you read aloud the more skillful you will become.

Vocal variety exercises using extant texts'

1. Speak this extract from Charles Dickens's *A Tale of Two Cities*. Develop the contrast between the opposites with changes in vocal quality. Allow the voice to express the quality of contrasting words: wisdom, foolishness, belief, incredulity, good, evil etc. Use pitch changes to convey the antithesis.

    It was the best of times, it was the worst of times, it was the age
    of wisdom, it was the age of foolishness, it was the epoch of belief,
    it was the epoch of incredulity, it was the season of Light, it was the
    season of Darkness, it was the spring of hope, it was the winter of

despair, we had everything before us, we had nothing before us, we were all going direct to Heaven, we were all going direct the other way – in short, the period was so far like the present period, that some of its noisiest authorities insisted on its being received, for good or for evil, in the superlative degree of comparison only.

2. Speak the following extract. Allow the voice to convey the varying periods of time and the opposing actions: born/die, plant/pluck up, kill/heal etc.

To everything there is a season, and a time to every purpose under the heaven:
A time to be born, and a time to die; a time to plant, and a time to pluck up that which is planted;
A time to kill, and a time to heal; a time to break down, and a time to build up;
A time to weep, and a time to laugh; a time to mourn, and a time to dance;
A time to cast away stones, and a time to gather stones together; a time to embrace, and a time to refrain from embracing;
A time to get, and a time to lose; a time to keep, and a time to cast away;
A time to rend, and a time to sew; a time to keep silence, and a time to speak;
A time to love, and a time to hate; a time of war, and a time of peace.

From: Ecclesiastes 3, *King James Version* of The Bible.

3. Read the following extract and focus on distinguishing the antithesis between (poor/rich, base-born/noble subject/sovereign etc.).

It is virtue, yea virtue, gentlemen, that maketh gentlemen; that maketh the poor rich, the base-born noble, the subject a sovereign, the deformed beautiful, the sick whole, the weak strong, the most miserable most happy. There are two principal and peculiar gifts in the nature of man, knowledge and reason; the one commandeth, and the other obeyeth: these things neither the whirling wheel of fortune can change, neither the deceitful cavillings of worldlings separate, neither sickness abate, neither age abolish".

From: John Lyly, *Euphues, The Anatomy of Wit* (1578).

4. Try singing/chanting the Dickens text (p. 339) as if in an operetta. Notice how the vowels lengthen, speech becomes more melodious and range increases dramatically. It is always important to monitor breath support and capacity with song, and to avoid areas of tension or forcing of the voice. Alternatively, sing the words of the Dickens extract to any popular contemporary tune you know well.

5. Take the Dickens text exercise from song/chant into speech, trying to find a similarly melodious quality. Incorporate gesture and use this to aid vocalization. It may be appropriate to grade this exercise so that it has three distinct stages:

    (a) song/chant;
    (b) melodramatic speech with a song-/chant-like quality; and
    (c) speech with more melody than usual.

    NB: In all these exercises, control and capacity of breath is vital but any temptation to 'push' vocally must be resisted. Maintain easy relaxed and preferably playful voicing at all times. The following pages offer suggestions for working on extant speeches in order to exercise skills in public speaking. The exercise is also excellent for practicing vocal variety.

Making a speech

When working on your speech and when addressing public speaking issues in the classroom remember the following:

- Prepare well so that you feel confident.
- Research your audience and formulate your speech accordingly.
- Familiarize yourself with the space and lectern if you are using one.
- Assess the height and width of the room, the texture of the curtains and carpets, etc., as these will affect the acoustic.
- Rehearse your speech in the space so that you can hear how the acoustic works before you give your presentation.
- Ask for feedback on vocal levels.
- Insist on a sound level check if you are using a microphone.
- Welcome the surge of adrenaline. Don't be afraid of it, it is natural and you can use it positively.
- Avoid overly rapid breathing as this can add to your nervousness.
- Breathing out is important as we 'hold breath' in stressful situations.
- Make a positive entrance and hold your space.
- Connect with the audience by looking at all of them, making eye contact with some and smiling at them before you begin.
- Speak more slowly that you would in conversation as your audience needs time to hear, decode, understand, and respond to your words.
- Move confidently and deliberately in a relaxed manner, rather than shuffling the feet or fidgeting.
- If something goes wrong, correct it and move on. Audiences do not mind vulnerability. In fact it can win them over.
- Consider the way posture or body language might be perceived.
- Finish your speech on a definite note so that the audience knows when to clap, avoid 'fizzling or fading out' as it confuses the audience.
- Answer questions in a firm and friendly way and if you do not know the answer, simply say so.
- Remain physically and vocally confident until you have exited the room.

For many, making a speech is extremely stressful. Changing the focus from you to your audience is often a positive way of reducing self-consciousness and fear.

These outward focus suggestions may help:

- Focus on the message and your audience rather than your situation, and the situation will become less intimidating.
- Greet your audience with a smile, it will put you and the audience at ease.
- Make confident eye contact with members of your audience, don't look over their heads or at the floor.
- Your desire to share your information is paramount.
- Your audience wants to hear what you have to say.
- They also want you to succeed.
- Looking after their needs will shift the focus from your own.
- Put them at their ease by being physically confident.
- Be loud enough for them to hear you.
- Be slow enough for them to understand you.
- Allow the voice to be varied and interesting so that the audience is engaged.
- Emphasize the important information and the details they need to remember.
- Avoid emphasizing with stress only; use pause, inflection, and pitch to make significant words and phrases more easily remembered.
- Attempt to make the formal occasion relaxed and conversational so that your audience can feel they are involved in a conversation.
- Include elements of rhetoric (the art of persuasion) that connect with your audience, such as humour, empathy, and logic.
- Smiling not only breaks down barriers and helps the audience and the speaker to relax and engage, it also 'brightens' the vocal quality and allows for greater vocal range.

Structure of speeches

The way in which a speech is structured is very important but is not the subject of this book. The Further Reading section at the end of the chapter offers suggestions for helpful sources. Here are some examples of extant speeches that will provide the opportunity to practice skills in vocal variety and speechmaking. Working with well structured speeches provides the reader with some insight into the power of rhetoric.

Additional exercise material

Rhetoric is not a principal concern of this book, but as public speaking forms a significant part of many educators' working lives, here is some exercise material. There are many excellent specialist books on the subject, and they offer more detailed information on the classical art of persuasion, which is as important today as it was in Ancient Greece and Rome. Useful titles can be found in the Suggested Reading section at the end of this chapter.

In the examples that follow, notice how the speaker appeals to the audience. They may engage the audience by promoting their good character and ethics (*ethos*), or by influencing the audience through a shared frame of mind (*pathos*), or by applying logic to the argument and providing evidence to prove their case (*logos*).

There are many more rhetorical devices worth noting and using, such as repetition, the use of antithesis, alliteration, assonance, lists (often three point lists) puzzles, pause, and the use of simile and metaphor etc. A speaker can also ask a question of the audience and then go on to provide an answer.

Notice the structure of the speeches, which, in their simplest form, much as an essay or a story, have an introduction, body and conclusion. The much quoted Aristotelian advice 'Tell them what you are going to tell them, tell them, then tell them what you said' clearly underlines the need for repetition. Words, when spoken not read, need to be conveyed with conviction. If the speaker conveys the message clearly with passion, commitment and generosity, allowing the voice to convey these qualities through vocal variety and effective communication, the audience will listen and become involved.

In this first speech, Susan B. Anthony creates empathy with her audience by addressing them as 'Friends and fellow citizens'. She states the charge and then sets out her intention to prove it false. She states that she is simply 'exercising her rights' under the National Constitution and goes on to quote it. Notice how her use of antithesis builds her argument. Consider the ways in which this argument can be conveyed by vocal variety through changes in inflection, nuance, pitch and pause. In the subsequent speeches, look for similar styles and structures.

1. *Susan B. Anthony,* On Women's Right to Vote *(1873)*

    Friends and fellow citizens: I stand before you tonight under indictment for the alleged crime of having voted at the last presidential election, without having a lawful right to vote. It shall be my work this evening to prove to you that in thus voting, I not only committed no crime, but, instead, simply exercised my citizen's rights, guaranteed to me and all United States citizens by the National Constitution, beyond the power of any state to deny.

    The preamble of the Federal Constitution says:

    "We, the people of the United States, in order to form a more perfect union, establish justice, insure domestic tranquillity, provide for the common defence, promote the general welfare, and secure the blessings of liberty to ourselves and our posterity, do ordain and establish this Constitution for the United States of America".

    It was we, the people; not we, the white male citizens; nor yet we, the male citizens; but we, the whole people, who formed the Union. And we formed it, not to give the blessings of liberty, but to secure them; not to the half of ourselves and the half of our posterity, but to the whole people – women as well as men. And it is a downright mockery to talk to women of their enjoyment of the blessings of liberty while they are denied the use of the only means of securing them provided by this democratic-republican government - the ballot.

2.   *Emmeline Pankhurst,* Freedom or Death *(1913)*

We women, in trying to make our case clear, always have to make as part of our argument, and urge upon men in our audience the fact – a very simple fact – that women are human beings . . .

We were called militant, and we were quite willing to accept the name. We were determined to press this question of the enfranchisement of women to the point where we were no longer to be ignored by the politicians.

We wear no mark; we belong to every class; we permeate every class of the community from the highest to the lowest; and so you see in the woman's civil war the dear men of my country are discovering it is absolutely impossible to deal with it: you cannot locate it, and you cannot stop it.

3.   *Queen Elizabeth I,* Speech to the Troops at Tilbury *(1588)*

My loving people

We have been persuaded by some that are careful of our safety, to take heed how we commit ourselves to armed multitudes, for fear of treachery; but I assure you I do not desire to live to distrust my faithful and loving people. Let tyrants fear. I have always so behaved myself that, under God, I have placed my chiefest strength and safeguard in the loyal hearts and good-will of my subjects; and therefore I am come amongst you, as you see, at this time, not for my recreation and disport, but being resolved, in the midst and heat of the battle, to live and die amongst you all; to lay down for my God, and for my kingdom, and my people, my honour and my blood, even in the dust.

I know I have the body of a weak, feeble woman; but I have the heart and stomach of a king, and of a king of England too, and think foul scorn that Parma or Spain, or any prince of Europe, should dare to invade the borders of my realm; to which rather than any dishonour shall grow by me, I myself will take up arms, I myself will be your general, judge, and rewarder of every one of your virtues in the field.

I know already, for your forwardness you have deserved rewards and crowns; and we do assure you on a word of a prince, they shall be duly paid. In the mean time, my lieutenant general shall be in my stead, than whom never prince commanded a more noble or worthy subject; not doubting but by your obedience to my general, by your concord in the camp, and your valour in the field, we shall shortly have a famous victory over these enemies of my God, of my kingdom, and of my people.

4. *Napoleon Bonaparte,* Farewell to the Old Guard *(1814)*

Soldiers of my Old Guard: I bid you farewell. For twenty years I have constantly accompanied you on the road to honour and glory. In these latter times, as in the days of our prosperity, you have invariably been models of courage and fidelity. With men such as you our cause could not be lost; but the war would have been interminable; it would have been civil war, and that would have entailed deeper misfortunes on France.

I have sacrificed all of my interests to those of the country.

I go, but you, my friends, will continue to serve France. Her happiness was my only thought. It will still be the object of my wishes. Do not regret my fate; if I have consented to survive, it is to serve your glory. I intend to write the history of the great achievements we have performed together. Adieu, my friends. Would I could press you all to my heart.

5. *Edmund Burke,* On the Death of Marie Antoinette *(1793)*

. . . little did I dream that I should have lived to see such disasters fallen upon her, in a nation of gallant men, in a nation of men of honour, and of cavaliers! I thought ten thousand swords must have leaped from their scabbards, to avenge even a look that threatened her with insult.

But the age of chivalry is gone; that of sophisters, economists, and calculators has succeeded, and the glory of Europe is extinguished forever. Never, never more, shall we behold that generous loyalty to rank

and sex, that proud submission, that dignified obedience, that subordi-
nation of the heart, which kept alive, even in servitude itself, the spirit
of an exalted freedom! The unbought grace of life, the cheap defence of
nations, the nurse of manly sentiment and heroic enterprise is gone. It
is gone, that sensibility of principle, that chastity of honour, which felt
a stain like a wound, which inspired courage whilst it mitigated feroc-
ity, which ennobled whatever it touched, and under which vice itself
lost half its evil, by losing all its grossness.

6. *Sojourner Truth,* Ain't I A Woman *(ca. 1851)*

Well, children, where there is so much racket there must be something
out of kilter. I think that 'twixt the negroes of the South and the women
at the North, all talking about rights, the white men will be in a fix
pretty soon. But what's all this here talking about?

That man over there says that women need to be helped into car-
riages, and lifted over ditches, and to have the best place everywhere.
Nobody ever helps me into carriages, or over mud-puddles, or gives me
any best place! And ain't I a woman? Look at me! Look at my arm!
I have ploughed and planted, and gathered into barns, and no man
could head me! And ain't I a woman? I could work as much and eat as
much as a man – when I could get it – and bear the lash as well! And
ain't I a woman? I have borne thirteen children, and seen most all sold
off to slavery, and when I cried out with my mother's grief, none but
Jesus heard me! And ain't I a woman?

Then they talk about this thing in the head; what's this they call it?
[member of audience whispers, "intellect"] That's it, honey. What's that
got to do with women's rights or negroes' rights? If my cup won't hold
but a pint, and yours holds a quart, wouldn't you be mean not to let me
have my little half measure full?

Then that little man in black there, he says women can't have as
much rights as men, 'cause Christ wasn't a woman! Where did your

Christ come from? Where did your Christ come from? From God and
a woman! Man had nothing to do with Him.

If the first woman God ever made was strong enough to turn the
world upside down all alone, these women together ought to be able to
turn it back, and get it right side up again! And now they is asking to
do it, the men better let them.

Obliged to you for hearing me, and now old Sojourner ain't got
nothing more to say.

7.   *Mark Antony from William Shakespeare,* Julius Caesar

Notice how in this last well known speech from Shakespeare the character
Mark Antony uses many of the same devices, particularly antithesis and repetition. His seeming flattery of Brutus allows his to achieve his goal without
alienating the crowd.

Friends, Romans, countrymen, lend me your ears;
I come to bury Caesar, not to praise him.
The evil that men do lives after them;
The good is oft interred with their bones;
So let it be with Caesar. The noble Brutus
Hath told you Caesar was ambitious:
If it were so, it was a grievous fault,
And grievously hath Caesar answer'd it.
Here, under leave of Brutus and the rest--
For Brutus is an honourable man;
So are they all, all honourable men--
Come I to speak in Caesar's funeral.
He was my friend, faithful and just to me:
But Brutus says he was ambitious;
And Brutus is an honourable man.
He hath brought many captives home to Rome
Whose ransoms did the general coffers fill:
Did this in Caesar seem ambitious?

When that the poor have cried, Caesar hath wept:
Ambition should be made of sterner stuff:
Yet Brutus says he was ambitious;
And Brutus is an honourable man.
You all did see that on the Lupercal
I thrice presented him a kingly crown,
Which he did thrice refuse: was this ambition?
Yet Brutus says he was ambitious;
And, sure, he is an honourable man.
I speak not to disprove what Brutus spoke,
But here I am to speak what I do know.
You all did love him once, not without cause:
What cause withholds you then, to mourn for him?
O judgment! thou art fled to brutish beasts,
And men have lost their reason. Bear with me;
My heart is in the coffin there with Caesar,
And I must pause till it come back to me.

Act III, scene II

Vocal Preparation Routines

The following can be used by individuals or adapted for classes.

Routine 1: floor exercises

1. Spine: lengthen the spine. Imagine that you are able gently to separate the vertebrae by moving the head away from the shoulders and the hips from the ribs. Broaden the back by imagining that you can widen the shoulder girdle. Gently press the shoulders into the floor, then release. Feel that you are longer and broader than you were.

2. Jaw and tongue: imagine that the jaw hangs off the skull. Feel the space between the teeth. Stretch the tongue out of the mouth, release it, and allow it to slip back to a position where it loosely touches the

lower front teeth. Clench the teeth, release, and then release a second time. Repeat the exercise three times.

3.   Scalp: release the muscles of the face and scalp. Imagine that you are wearing a tennis sweatband across the forehead. Using the muscles of the face and head, imagine pushing it off the top of the head.

4.   Neck: release the back of the neck by lengthening it. It sometimes helps to push the head gently into the floor; feel the tension, then release it. Gently move the head from the left to the right shoulder. Bring the head back to a central position.

5.   Breath:

(a)   Place one hand on the centre of the body, in the region of the navel. The most extensive breathing activity should ideally happen below the sternum and in the area of the abdomen and lower ribs. At best, the movement you feel as the breath displaces the muscles of the abdomen should be below the navel. Sigh out a feeling of being bored. Notice how the breath returns on its own. Sigh out a feeling of relief; again notice how the breath returns on its own.

(b)   Breathing out, notice how the hand sinks down towards the floor. Feel the breath pass over the lips on a gentle /fff/. When you have emptied the lungs, pause and wait until you feel the need for breath. Do not resist it, simply allow the breath to return and notice how the hand on the body rises up towards the ceiling and the lower ribs move upwards and outwards to allow the breath to fill the space below the sternum. The shoulders, neck, and upper chest need not be involved.

(c)   Repeat the exercise above breathing out on the sound /sh/. Notice that the breath is used up more quickly on this sound.

(d)   In your head, count to five on an /s/ as you breathe out. Make sure that you keep the neck and jaw loose. Do not worry about the quality of the /s/. On the next outgoing breath, count in your head to six, and so on. Do not feel that it is important to reach a high number. If you get tense and tight in attempting to do so you have defeated the object of the exercise. Notice that the ribs as well as the muscles under the hand are active in releasing the breath.

(e)   Now feeling very loose (the idea of being pleasantly drunk helps) turn the outgoing breath into sound and voice the sound /mah/. Build a feeling of vibration in the 'mask' of the face on /mmm/ before opening on to the vowel.

(f)   Do the same using /nah/, /vah/, and /zah/.

(g)   Begin to vary both the pitch and the vowel so that you produce a combination of sounds beginning with /n/, e.g. /noh/, /naw/, /nay/, /now/; do the same using /v/ and /z/.

Routine 2: working in a chair

1.   Begin by sitting in an upright chair (such as one commonly used in classrooms). Make sure that you find it comfortable. Sit with both 'sitting bones' firmly on the seat. Avoid sitting on one buttock only. Lengthen the spine from the coccyx to the skull. Avoid over-correction and hollowing of the lower back. Feel that the spine is free and flexible. Use the Alexander Technique image of a water fountain spouting up through the spine. Let the head be balanced on the top of the spine. Make small movements to the muscles of the neck so as to move the head minimally. No large movements of the head should occur. The feeling to work for is that of the marionette's head, loose but not floppy. Let the jaw feel as if it 'hangs off the head'. Let the tongue feel loose and free in the mouth with the tongue tip touching the lower front teeth.

2.   Take the chair and sit back to front on it, so that you can lean over the backrest. This will open up the vertebrae in the lower spine and, as long as you release and 'let go' of the shoulders, it is a good position for breathing. You can put your head on your folded arms across the back of the chair.

3.   If possible, ask someone to place their thumbs on your spine with the fingers splayed around the lower ribs. This will allow both of you to

feel the expansion of the ribs when you breathe in. The movement will result in the thumbs moving away from the spine.

4. Set up a steady rhythm of breathing in and out. Work on breathing in to a count of three and then out to three, then in to a count of three and out to four, and in to three and out to five. As the breath leaves the body, feel it pass between the teeth and lips in a gentle /fff/. Never get competitive and try to get up to a high count because this leads to breath-holding and creates more tension than it releases.

5. On the outgoing breath begin to introduce an effortless /vvv/ by simply turning the breathed /fff/ into sound. Feel the vibrations on the lips and teeth and in the mask of the face. If you feel discomfort in the larynx or tension in the back of the neck, you are working too hard.

6. In this position speak a few lines of text. A traditional rhyme, words of a song, or simply count from one to ten.

Routine 3: exercises in connecting resonators

(To be done after Routine 1 or 2, or after doing the resonance exercises.)

Sliding and gliding

Use the whole body and move whenever possible during these exercises.

1. Sirening: using the sound /n/ (and imitating the noise of a police siren) describe a vocal circle that begins between the shoulder blades and 'slide' the sound over the top of the head and face. Keeping the sound moving, return to the starting point along an imaginary circular trajectory. This should be easy as long as you keep it playful and do not try to push. You will not hurt the voice in this way. The same can be done with the /ng/ sound (in song) and the /m/, /v/, and /z/.

2. Slide: stretching up with hands in the air, allow the spine to bend over, one vertebra at a time, until you are bent over at the waist. As you do so make the sound of a vowel, such as /oo/, /ay/, /aw/, or /ah/. Make the vowel last as long as the journey from the extended

stretch to the bent spine. This exercise can be done in reverse, starting the sound on the floor and sliding it upwards. Some people find this direction easier; others find it more difficult. Eventually both will be possible. If you find the onset of the vowel difficult precede it with an /m/.

3. Bowling: using the arm to bowl, imagine the ball is the sound /m/ and as it leaves your hand lift the sound up and over the space almost in an arc. Open to the vowel /ah/ halfway through the arc and sustain the sound until it 'lands' on the ground. Do this in slow motion so that it blends from the /m/ into the /ah/ smoothly as it arcs through the air.

4. Glide from chest to mouth: make an /ah/, producing chest resonance. Feel the vibration by placing your hand on your chest. Make an /aw/, being aware of the resonance in the mouth. Notice how the lips form a megaphone shape.

5. Begin by patting the chest while sounding /mah/ – feel the vibrations. Glide the /ah/ vowel into an /aw/ in the mouth, slurring from one sound to another, e.g. /mah … aw/.

6. Repeat the exercise beginning with the /aw/ resonating in the mouth and then glide this sound upwards into an /ee/. The glide from the /aw/ to the /ee/ should be relaxed and effortless, and the overall balance of one sound moving from one space to another should be maintained. In all these exercises the smooth continuum of sound is worked for, and any feeling of pushed or strangulated sounds should be avoided. If a 'crack' in the flow of sound develops, just go slowly back over that area in the range. Using the hand or arm to describe the movement is often an effective aid to developing flexibility of the voice.

7. Fire engine/ambulance siren: using /ng … ah/ /ng … ah/ /ng … ah/, create the movement between head and chest resonance. This exercise explores the vocal range and extends the extremes of pitch and resonance. The dual-pitch siren is used for different vehicles in

different cities, so the title of this exercise may not be correct for everyone, but can be adapted.

8. Slurring and singing: using a piece of text (just a few lines), slur the voice drunkenly and smoothly through the whole range. Try a line sung to a made-up tune. Speak it to that tune. Reduce the tune but keep the movement in the voice.

It is important to 'play' and not to strive for perfection because this usually results in creating tension rather than releasing it.

Routine 4: exercises for primary classes
Exercises for teachers and learners

1. Ask the class to stretch and yawn like a cat, not forgetting to stretch the spine, fingers, and toes.

2. Everyone should wrinkle up the face so as to pull the ugliest face possible. Relax. Then smile as widely as possible. Relax.

3. Stretch the tongue out as far as possible as if 'pulling tongues'. Relax.

4. Blow through the lips like a horse in order to loosen the mouth area. Relax.

5. Imagine the class is playing tennis. To begin with, use the sound /b/ as the ball and everyone uses an imaginary tennis racquet to hit the /b/. The first part of the exercise is bouncing the /b/ on the racquet using short staccato sounds. The second part of the exercise is to lengthen the stroke so that the /b/ develops into a /bah/ and travels a distance. The distance should be specified, e.g., 'Let the /bah/ land on the floor at the other end of the line/classroom/hall'. Sometimes these exercises are best done in slow motion. The consonant /d/ can be similarly used and developed into /dah/ for the second part of the exercise.

6. Use 'mirroring' exercises in pairs to warm up the muscles of the face and the tongue. This requires the pair to work together and to focus on the specific muscles of speech. It is also fun and breaks down barriers.

7. If possible, teach the class a few phrases in a foreign language so as to allow them to take up vocal and verbal positions not encountered in English or in the mother tongue. Explore and enjoy these different sounds and positions.

8. Create sounds that require pitch change and wide range such as sirens, revving cars, planes, bird calls, and cats miaowing.

9. Blow up the cheeks and with the fingers pop them. Blow raspberries. Make the noise of a motorbike to the sound /brmmmm/ and of a speedboat to the sound /vrmmmm/.

10. Ask the class to explore the dynamics of these words: as they say the first word they should use the body to discover the innate energy (no physical contact should take place). Ask them to:

   - pull a light weight;
   - push a heavy load uphill;
   - twist a tight lid off a jar;
   - tug at a trapped rope;
   - bash two dustbin lids together;
   - bend a piece of pipe;
   - bounce on a trampoline;
   - dig a hole in the ground;
   - dive off a high diving board;
   - dab paint on the wall;
   - wring out a wet towel; or
   - wriggle out of a tight space.

11. It is important to bring the exercises together in connected speech and to strive for expressive communication. There is wonderful contemporary verse or prose that is suitable for this.

To conclude this exercise session, ask the group to speak the following extract focusing on the muscularity and energy of the words as well as releasing the rhythm:

357

On the top of the Crumpetty Tree
The Quangle Wangle sat,
But his face you could not see,
On account of his Beaver Hat.
For his Hat was a hundred and two feet wide,
With ribbons and bibbons on every side
And bells, and buttons, and loops, and lace,
So that nobody ever could see the face
Of the Quangle Wangle Quee.

From: Edward Lear, *The Quangle Wangle's Hat*

Routine 5: exercises for secondary classes
Exercises for teachers and students

1. Standing, ask the class to follow you in stretching up through the right-hand side. Take the arm above the head and over to the left side. The greatest extension is felt when the heel of the hand is used in the stretch. Now do the same with the left arm, taking it up and then over to the right. Make the class aware of the movement of the ribcage in the stretch.

2. Ask the class to stand as badly as they possibly can. This usually involves standing with the weight on one leg, and the head and shoulders slumping forward. Often the arms will be folded across the chest and generally, there will be a reduction of space between the hips and lower ribs, making easy breathing, centred in the diaphragmatic and lower rib area, difficult.

   The second part of this exercise is to ask them to correct the posture, so that they draw themselves up and out of the slumped position, readjusting their weight so that it is equally distributed across both feet. The spine will be long, the chest open and the head easily balanced on top of the spine. Once the class recognizes the difference between 'bad and 'good' alignment, they can take it in turns to stand badly so that a partner can physically change their posture by moving them into a more open and more aligned position. This exercise can be done as 'puppets' with quite young children, e.g., A is the puppet, B the puppeteer who rearranges the puppet's posture.

3. The class should now divide into pairs, and take it in turns to do the following exercises. One of the pair monitors and feeds back information to the partner actively involved in the exercise, a very important task. Feedback should be about the physicality observed and the level of tension monitored. Partner A stands in front of partner B and tries to release all tension from the shoulder area. Partner B then lifts the shoulder girdle of A and reports on how much, if any, resistance is encountered. Generally, A will either hold the shoulders down or assist in raising them. The aim is to do neither, but rather to release the shoulders so that they can be moved by B. This is best achieved by attempting to isolate the shoulders and giving up all control over them. If the shoulders are locked they will be difficult to move; if, however, A is successful in isolating them, B will feel that they are heavy but loose. Feedback is very useful here because it begins to raise awareness of just how much tension is being held in the shoulder girdle. Change over so that A becomes the monitor and B does the exercise.

4. Once the shoulders have been released, a similar exercise is done with the arms. Partner A stands or sits with the arms hanging loosely by the sides. B lifts A's arm as A attempts to release the muscles, making the arm fully pliable and flexible and under the control of B. The temptation again is for A to control the arm, particularly when the arm is raised. When the arm is dropped by B, the arm may remain in 'mid-air', illustrating that the muscles retain tension. Change over and repeat, remembering the importance of feedback. The difficulty of releasing habitually held tension in the shoulders and the arms should not be under-estimated, but this exercise is fun.

5. The class should stand, with knees unlocked and spine long. They should become aware of the way in which the head balances on the

top of the spine and, releasing the jaw, should gently allow the head to nod in a small 'yes' gesture (up and down) and then in a 'no' gesture from side to side. Movements should be loose but minimal.

6. Move the head towards the right shoulder and, using the nose as a pencil, 'draw' straight lines from floor to ceiling while travelling towards the left shoulder. The action here should again be one of fluidity and ease rather than of high energy. The muscles of the neck will feel the lengthening effect of the exercise. It is very important that the jaw should not be clenched.

7. In pairs again, A should stand in front of B. B places his or her hands around the lower ribs of A with the thumbs resting on either side of the spine. Beginning with A breathing out, B should notice how much the lower ribs decrease in width as breath is exhaled. The A group should be told to wait gently until they feel the need to breathe, and then both A and B should notice how the breath replenishes and how, as it does so, B's hands on A's ribs move outward and the thumbs move away from the spine. Repeat, changing over A and B. It is important for A to feed back information about the movement as it occurs.

8. Ask the whole class to pat their chests as they release the sound /mah/. They should be encouraged to feel the vibrations in the chest. Class members should imagine drawing the letter /m/. They should use the hand slowly to describe the letter as the voice follows, thereby opening up and exploring the range. They can then describe a circle using /nnnnnn/ while drawing the circle at the same time. In all these exercises it is important to feel the vibrations rather than listening to the sound.

9. Blow up the cheeks and with the fingers pop them. Blow raspberries. Make the noise of a motorbike to the sound /brmmmm/ and of a speedboat to the sound /vrmmmm/.

10. Using gibberish, ask members of the class to improvise a few lines in a made-up language and let the class repeat it. The object here is not

to produce perfect sounds, but to explore a different usage of sound sequences.

11.   Select a short passage of text that has energized language and let the class explore this together. Do not be concerned about analysing meaning; simply encourage exploration and enjoyment in the speaking of the words. Meaning will gradually evolve.

> *Blow, blow thou winter wind,*
> *Thou art not so unkind*
> *As man's ingratitude;*
> *Thy tooth is not so keen,*
> *Because thou art not seen,*
> *Although thy breath be rude.*
> *Heigh Ho! Sing, Heigh Ho! unto the green holly*
> *Most friendship is feigning, most loving mere folly:*
> *Then, heigh ho! the holly!*
> *This life is most jolly.*

From: William Shakespeare, *As You Like It* (Act II, scene vii)

Routine 6: short warm-up (i)

This warm-up uses some of the exercises already described in this chapter. Some warming up can be done quite inconspicuously in the bus or the car, or on the train.

Loosening the body

1.   Gently push the shoulder blades together and feel the opening of the front of the chest as you do so. Do this three times.

2.   Lift the shoulders slightly and then release them. Do this three or four times.

3.   Using two fingers of the right hand gently push the chin into the neck and feel the stretch of the muscles down the back of the neck. Do this three times.

4.   Imagine that the head is balanced on the top of the spine on a greasy ball-bearing.

5.   Move the head very smoothly and easily in a nodding 'Yes' motion.

Loosening the jaw

Checking the level of tension in the jaw is always recommended.

1.   Take the hands up to the cheekbones and gently stroke the jaw downwards allowing the strap muscle to release and lengthen.

2.   Imagine that the jaw is heavy and let its weight carry the jaw downward. Feel the separation of the teeth. Monitor whether or not the teeth are clenched; if so release the strap muscle.

Breathing out

1.   Sigh out to the count of five on an /ff/. When the lungs empty, simply allow them to refill.

2.   Sigh out to a count of six on an /ss/. Repeat the refill process.

3.   Sigh out to a count of seven on a /th/. Repeat the refill process.

4.   Sigh out to a count of eight on a /sh/. Repeat the refill process.

If you are in a private space (the car is ideal, as long as it is not overheated and your shoulders and neck are not locked in a state of tension as a result of traffic jams) you can begin to voice on the outgoing sigh.

5.   Sing out to a count of seven on /mmmmm/.

6.   Sing out to a count of eight on /vvvvvv/.

7.   Sing out to a count of nine on /zzzzz/.

Count in your head while you voice the sounds. If you prefer to use numbers instead of sounds you can count from one to five, then start again from one and add a number until you reach your limit. Always be aware of tension in the muscles of the neck when you sound, particularly as you come to the end of the breath capacity.

Moving the voice

1. Describe a line from the floor to the ceiling using a trilled /r/. At first you may find that you cannot sustain the line of breath and sound, but with practice you soon will.

2. Hum any familiar tune. Purse the lips as you hum and maintain space between the upper and lower teeth in order to encourage the voice to be placed forward on the lips and in the mask of the face.

3. Siren from your lowest note to your highest note using the sound /n/ or /ng/.

Vowels

It is important to explore the length of vowels, e.g., /heat/, /he/, and /heal/ all contain the same vowel /ee/ but, depending on the sound that follows, the length of the vowel is altered.

1. Try this sequence: /mmmm aw/ /mmmm oh/ /mmmm ee/, sustaining the vowel.

2. Feel that the /mmm/ brings the voice forward on to the lips and that the vowels are free, forward and not held in the throat.

3. Try working with /h/ in front of the vowels, e.g., /h-ah/ /h-ay/ /h-aw/.

Lips and tongue

1. Purse the lips and then circle them: beginning at the right-hand corner of your mouth, take the lips down toward your chin, round to the left-hand corner and then up to the nose and back to the starting point. Reverse the action.

2. Repeat the same exercise with the tongue and make sure that you stretch it and attempt to describe the full circle. Avoid missing out any section of the circle.

Consonants

When exercising the consonants it is important to feel the muscularity of the sounds.

1. The best way to exercise these sounds is to speak a short passage of verse that includes a plethora of consonants.

    The Jeweller sold the jewels to the judicious Duke of Donnington.
    Who displayed his diamonds to the jury?
    The Duke then fought a dual over Julia which he duly lost as he slipped on the dew.

2. Exercising complex combinations is demanding; try these clusters:

pests	*posts*	*roasts*
hosts	*masts*	*priests*
firsts	*chests*	*lists*
thrusts	*boasts*	*toasts*

3. Sounds move from voiced /dzh/ (*hedge*) to voiceless /tsh/ (*church*). These sounds are a combination of /d+zh/ and /t+sh/.

    Hedge sparrows hatch eggs in church hedgerows.
    Jumping jellybeans are enjoyed by cheerful gentlemen.
    Jade, Chelsea, John and Chester took the challenge to judge the Chiltern high jump.
    Generally etching is a June and July enjoyment in Chingford.

4. To end, speak this extract from Shakespeare enjoying the images he creates with both vowels and consonants:

    Full fathom five thy father lies,
    Of his bones are coral made;
    Those are the pearls that were his eyes;
    Nothing of him that doth fade,
    But doth suffer a sea-change
    Into something rich and strange.

    From: William Shakespeare, *The Tempest* (Act I, scene i)

Routine 7: short warm up (ii)

Stretches

1. If you have space do a full body stretch. Reach arms above the head and walk them towards the ceiling to open up the ribs.
2. Stretch the right arm over the head to the left side, leading with the heel of the hand.
3. Repeat on the other side.
4. Clasp hands behind you to open up the sternum. Hold. Release.
5. Clasp the hands in front of the body and reach forward opening up the space between the shoulder blades. Hold. Release.
6. Lift shoulders to ears. Hold. Release.
7. Push shoulders down towards the floor and away from the ears. Hold. Release.
8. Squat to open up the hips and lower back – let the breath drop down so you can feel the muscles move against your legs.

If you don't have space to do a full stretch, exercises 3 and 4 can be done sitting down. Exercise 5 can be done sitting in a chair and dropping the head and arms between the knees.

Face muscles

1. Smile widely. Hold. Release. Repeat five times.
2. Scrunch up the face. Hold. Release.
3. Stretch the face with the tongue stretched out fully and eyes wide open. Hold. Release slowly.
4. Purse the lips to look like a trumpet fish. Smile widely. Repeat five times.
5. Rabbit face lift/wriggle upper lip and nose.
6. Blow up cheeks. Pop with fingers. Repeat five times.
7. Release jaw by stretching lower jaw in front of upper jaw.
8. Place tongue tip behind lower front teeth and bulk tongue outwards. Feel the stretch in the tongue and the jaw hinge.

Breath place hands around the waist

1. Working up and down the scale:

    - Blow through lips on a /b/.
    - Blow through lips on a /p/.
    - Blow through lips on a /brrr/.
    - Blow through lips on a /prrr/.

2. Connect with the deep lower muscles of the back and abdomen on::

    - The /f/ sound. Repeat three times.
    - Repeat /v/ three times.
    - Repeat /sh/ three times.
    - Repeat /zh/ three times.
    - Repeat /b...zh/ three times, moving from the /b/ to the /zh/ sounds.

    Become aware of the muscular activity in the low abdominal muscles and muscles in the back.

3. Using the nasal sound /n/, draw small circles. Involve your hand to describe the circle. Place the sound forward in the mask of the face and feel the vibrations. Repeat on /m/ allowing the size of the circle to grow with each circle. Repeat with /ng/.

Sliding and gliding

1. Using /ng/ let the voice describe geometric shapes.
2. Gently tap the chest with your fist to establish resonance on a sustained /hah/.
3. Add a suggestion of innuendo to this and let the sound slide into the head. (Imagine teasing a friend, suggesting you know something about them. It helps to let the face become involved.)

Aim to support the sound from the chest into the mask of the face.

Articulation

1. Lips:

    B-A-B Bab.
    B-E-B Beb.
    Bab Beb.
    B-I-B Bib.
    bab beb bib.
    B-O-B Bob.
    bab beb bib bob.
    B-U-B Bub.
    bab beb bib bob bub.
    Mumble, mumble, mumble.
    Murmur, murmur, murmur.
    Betty Botter bought some butter, but she said 'this butter's bitter'.

2. Front of the tongue:

    Particularly tactile.
    Particular tactility.
    Dottie's dainty titbits, the delightfully vitaminized teatime dainty,
      Delicately wrapped and definitely insulated with double thicknesses of
      damp deterrent tinfoil. Do you doubt us? Then there's only one thing to
      do – try Dotty's titbits today!

3. Back of the tongue:

    /k-ga/ /k-ga/ /k-ga/.
    Gargle with gerkins (repeat five times).
    /ng-ah/ /ng-ah/ /ng-ah/ (move from the nasalized /ng/ to the non-
      nasal vowel /ah/).

    Speak this sentence savouring the nasal consonants but placing the
    vowels forward in the mouth.

    Walking along singing songs and banging gongs.

4.   Dexterity:

Pad kid.
Poured curd.
Pulled cod (repeat five times).
Unique New York (repeat five times).

5.   Clusters:

Psssst, kitty, kitty, kitty!
Psst! shhhhh! (repeat five times).
/Oos-kit/, /aws-kit/, /ays-kit/, /ees-kit/.
Lauren Lee, Lauren Lee, Lauren Lee, Lauren Lee.
Falling walls, falling walls, falling walls, falling walls.
Putty battle.
Strudel noodle.
Mettle medal.
Middle muddle.
Kindly kitten.
Girdle garden.
The ghosts sat on the posts in their hosts.
Mists and frosts, mists and frosts
Acts and texts
Fifth, sixth, seventh, eighth, and twelfth

Conclusion

The context in which the exercises and strategies outlined in this book will be applied will be different for each individual, depending on the specific vocal demands that they encounter. The essential work undertaken by those who choose to teach, lecture or facilitate is reliant on a flexible and free vocal mechanism, and on the ability to convert thoughts and ideas into sounds, words and language. The fact that we take our voices so much for granted, and think about them only when they do not work effectively, is an indication of the general resilience of the voice and the synchronicity of thought and speech. When a problem does occur, it is often as a result of an increase in tension or stress, which alters the fine balance that usually exists between the production of voice and the effort levels required to achieve easy and effortless voicing.

Successful institutions answer the needs of both the students and staff. Raising the awareness of vocal needs among teachers, lecturers, facilitators, principals, governors, and those in charge of education authorities and educational training colleges, is therefore of paramount importance.

Voice problems can be successfully treated by specialists in the field of voice and it is important not to sacrifice a career that you love because of lack of specialist intervention. The help is out there. Go and get it.

This book will have been productive if, through its cocktail of early warning signs, anatomical information, strategies and exercises, it raises awareness of voice in general, promotes good vocal hygiene, and helps to steer teachers and professional voice users who are experiencing difficulty, towards the help that they need and can so easily find.

In industry and commerce, the focus is now on investment in staff in order to increase productivity; the focus in education must be on those who deliver it. Many educators who want to remain within the profession are unable to withstand the high levels of stress, stress that is often manifested in a voice problem, and move to less stressful careers.

It is our hope that this book may provide the necessary support, information and guidance to halt this inexorable process.

References and further reading

14 Inspiring Speeches by Indians You Can't Afford to Miss. Available at: <http://www.thebetterindia.com/11894/greatest-speeches-indians-most-inspirational/> [Accessed August 2017].

Anderson C. 2016. *TED Talks: The official TED guide to public speaking*. New York, NY: Houghton, Mifflin Harcourt.

Atkinson M. 2008. *Speech-Making and Presentation Made Easy*. London: Vermilion.

Atkinson M. 2004. *Lend Me Your Ears*. London: Vermilion.

BBC Speeches, Media Centre. Available at: <http://www.bbc.co.uk/mediacentre/speeches/> [Accessed August 2017].

BBC The Speaker. Available at: <http://www.bbc.co.uk/speaker/improve/> [Accessed August 2017].

Blaisdell B. 2000. *Great Speeches by Native Americans*. New York, NY: Dover Thrift.

Centre for Women and Democracy. *Political Speeches by Women*. Available at: <http://www.cfwd.org.uk/quotations-2/political-speeches-by-women> [Accessed August 2017].

Famous Speeches by Mahatma Ghandi. Available at: <http://www.mkgandhi.org/speeches/speechMain.htm> [Accessed August 2017].

Famous Women Speeches. Available at: <http://www.powerfulwords.info/speeches/Famous-Women-Speeches/> [Accessed August 2017].

Gallo C. 2014. *Talk Like Ted*. London: MacMillan.

The History Place. *Great Speeches Collection*. Available at: <http://www.historyplace.com/speeches/previous.htm> [Accessed August 2017].

Leith S. 2012. *You Talkin' to Me?* London: Profile Books.

McKenna SJ, Copeland L, Lamm LW. 1999. *The World's Greatest Speeches*. New York, NY: Dover Books.

Nelson Mandela Foundation. *Speeches*. Available at: <https://www.nelsonmandela.org/content/page/speeches> [Accessed August 2017].

Index

About the Authors

Dr. Stephanie Martin's career as a Speech and Language Therapist combined clinical practice, research, lecturing, supervision, and examining of MA and PhD projects, and writing. Her professional focus of interest lay in occupational voice disorders. She holds an MA in voice studies from the Royal Central School of Speech and Drama. Her doctoral research explored factors which have an impact on the vocal performance and vocal effectiveness of newly qualified teachers and lecturers. Stephanie is a Past-President of the British Voice Association and in 2005 she was awarded Fellowship of the Royal College of Speech and Language Therapists for research and teaching. Previous publications include *Working with Voice Disorders*, now in its second edition and *VIP: Voice Impact Profile*, both co-authored with Myra Lockhart.

Lyn Darnley began her career as a performer and presenter in theatre, television and radio. She is former Head of Voice, Text and Artist Development at the Royal Shakespeare Company. She was previously Head of Voice at Rose Bruford College. She has served as an external examiner on several courses. Her work and her doctoral research has focused on theatre voice and actor training. In 2008 she was awarded the Conference of Drama Schools medal for Services to Actor Training. Her work with teachers includes workshops for the RSC Education Department, University of Michigan and Teachers Groups in the USA and South Africa. She holds an MPhil from the University of Birmingham and a PhD from the University of London. Since retiring from the RSC she has continued to work as a consultant and runs workshops in the UK and abroad, focusing on classic text and presentation skills.

Stephanie and Lyn have been colleagues and friends for many years initially working together offering workshops for teachers under the auspices of the

Voice Research Society, Rose Bruford College, and various teacher asso-
ciations and education authorities. They have co-authored publications on
their work with the teachers' voice and have been invited speakers on this
subject at conferences in the UK and the USA.